# Spiritual Crisis

# Spiritual Crisis

*What's Really Behind Loss, Disease, and Life's Major Hurts*

Meredith L. Young-Sowers

STILLPOINT PUBLISHING

STILLPOINT PUBLISHING
Building a society that honors The Earth,
Humanity, and The Sacred in All Life.

For a free catalog or ordering information, write
Stillpoint Publishing, Box 640, Walpole, NH 03608, USA
or call
1-800-847-4014 TOLL FREE (Continental US, except NH)
1-603-756-9281 (Foreign and NH)

This book is manufactured in the United States of America.
Cover and text design by Karen Savary

Published by Stillpoint Publishing, Box 640,
Meetinghouse Road, Walpole, NH 03608

ISBN 0-913299-89-8

Library of Congress Cataloging in Publication Data

Young-Sowers, Meredith L. (Meredith Lady)
Spiritual crisis : what's really behind loss, disease, and
life's major hurts / Meredith L. Young-Sowers.
p. cm.
1. Self-actualization (Psychology) 2. Mind and body
3. Holism 4. Transpersonal psychology I. Title
BF637.S4Y68 1993
131—dc20                                    92-37833

1 3 5 7 9 8 6 4 2

# Dedication

To my parents, Jean and Hubert Woods,
for their unwavering love and support of my efforts
to commit to words the spiritual philosophy we share,
and their continued belief in the force of the human spirit
to emerge into a new era of relationship
with the God-force.

# Contents

# Acknowledgments

A book is a living thing that holds within its pages the Love, effort, and expertise of many dedicated people. I wish to thank:

- my dear friend and colleague in healing, Joanna Mott, who has allowed me to share in her healing and through our experience together to provide essential feedback on the effects of energy on the body, mind, feelings, and spirit.
- my husband, Errol, for his invaluable practical guidance, his emotional and spiritual support, and his supreme skill at editing my information, which often means bringing it out of the clouds and down to Earth.
- my lifelong friend and sister healer, Caroline Myss, whose insight, humor, and dedication to excellence

has helped me find and write from the depth and heart of my own wisdom.

- Stillpoint's senior editor, Dorothy Seymour, whose good sense and skillful pen have helped me in innumerable ways to craft this book into one that is easy to read yet effective and clear.
- my sister spiritual searcher, Gisela Rank, who as my assistant and an invaluable part of the Stillpoint staff, has lovingly edited and typed many versions of this book.
- Stillpoint's fine managing editor and my sister activist, Charmaine Wellington, whose depth and breadth of writing experience and expertise has helped me untangle many an involved premise.
- Stillpoint's magical Art Director, Karen Savary, for her beautiful cover and lovely book design.
- Stillpoint's newly found typesetter, Sally Nichols-Jacke, for her care and grace in translating this manuscript to the typed page.
- Karin Bell, Virginia Page, Philip Conover, Jessie Lynn Gentlewolf, and Joe Murphy of the Stillpoint staff, for their continued support through the many months of the writing of this book, even when it meant a greater workload for them.

# Preface

*Your Love will always make itself known through your words.*

This book may be for you, or it may be meant for you to give to someone you love. This book may also be meant for you to use in helping someone you love to heal.

Healing is the challenge that you or someone close to you faces now. If someone you love is in trouble, you may want to help but may not feel qualified, or you may feel the person in need hasn't asked you for assistance. In either case, you can help yourself and someone else to build renewed self-worth, awaken the blueprint of perfect health within the "body wisdom," reduce fear, restore Love, and open an inner pathway to a meaningful future.

In healing yourself, the first and most important thought as you begin your own healing journey is that now you are no longer alone—nor will you be alone in the weeks, months, or years ahead. Even though you may now be afraid and upset, you have begun an extraordinary and essential journey of inner awakening. This journey is the path to healing your loss, your physical pain, and your life.

The first step in healing yourself or others is to learn about the energy of Love that is the force of your spirit and the ways it can be harnessed to help you heal and become whole. Your spirit galvanizes intangible forces that you can call forth through your feelings, your thoughts, and your prayers to heal any loss, any physical disease, or any dysfunction.

Healing is a science based on Love and the use of energy. In healing we both give and receive the energy of life that comes from the God-force and also from our own bodies and emotions. When we are able to hold energy in our emotional and physical bodies, we can balance the upsetting, even the devastating, circumstances we encounter. But when in spiritual crisis our losses are too big and our troubles too great, we lose essential energy more quickly than we can replace it.

Love is both an emotion and a spiritual energy. Love is the basis for healing, because it unleashes our capacity to honor our lives as part of a larger, God-oriented system of life. When we accept that we are aligned with this force, we can draw strength and healing power through the energy bonds of this relationship. Spiritual energy awakens in our hearts the understanding that our difficult challenges are leading us toward, rather than away from, life health as we explore the spiritual dimension of our lives.

In order to heal ourselves or others, we are required to learn about energy: what creates it, what destroys it, and how it can be used and directed to heal ourselves and others. No one wants to be sick or miserable. And yet when we are in these situations, we tend to face life in a new way. We are forced to consider the quality of our lives, our spiritual beliefs, and whether or not we have a sincere desire to heal, change, and recover physically, emotionally, and spiritually. Healing begins when we accept that something of major significance is trying to be born within us, and our job is to stop resisting long enough to look at ourselves beneath the personality level. We can help ourselves, and we can help others, by using the gift that healers have always used: a compassionate, powerful belief in the God-force and an appreciation of Love as an energy.

When we are sick or afraid, we need the loving reassurance of others, including those involved in our care. We need to make our own decisions, to choose wisely from the smorgasbord of techniques and methods that can change disease to health or loss to recovery. We need to regain an enduring inner vitality or find it for the first time. We need to believe in our own goodness and in a future that may be difficult to envision.

This book is about healing and finding wholeness through Love and the acceptance of change. For you to help yourself or to help another person, no previous background in healing is required. We are all able to use Love to encourage inner and outer healing, but when we are in serious trouble and loss in spiritual crisis, we need those who care about us to support us in new ways.

Over the last ten years, I've worked with hundreds of people, and each has taught me something quite extraordinary. I've learned that the human spirit is tenacious beyond belief, and when it wills itself to stay within a human body, it often does. I've found that people can best direct their own treatment or recovery plans when they are encouraged to use their intuition and natural perception. Over and over again I've seen that Love commands more power than fear. I have held people who were preparing to die and others who were preparing to live, and I have felt humbled by their capacity to love beyond themselves, to learn from the most difficult situations, to change against all odds, and to heal their lives in ways they had not imagined possible.

You and the people who care about you can learn to use the energy of Love and the God-force to bring a new beginning into your lives. Your journey is primarily spiritual, even though your body and your emotions are the more obvious vehicles. If you believe that this is true, or if you are willing to proceed as if it were true, then turn the page, and let's begin an extraordinary journey that can heal your life.

MEREDITH L. YOUNG-SOWERS
Walpole, NH
November, 1992

*As you begin your healing journey,*
*the first and most important thing to remember*
*is that you are no longer alone—*
*you are linked through Love to the God-force ,*
*and as you draw on this powerful energy*
*you are able to heal your pain*
*and heal your life.*

# 1 Healing Begins By Trusting the Process of Spiritual Change

*You have a future that is meant to be filled with Love and community even though you don't see it or can't even imagine it.*

Our lives are like spinning tops. We've been spinning for many years, only now the spin is changing, and the orbits of that spin, our lives, are wobbling. This is because we are no longer centered around our inner truth: the remembrance that it is our souls, our capacity to love, that is our basis for life. We've pushed our limits, reaching too far from our centers, and now we feel loss, fear, anxiety, or disease. It is time for a change.

Our personal spiritual crisis is part of a much larger spiritual crisis that is occurring on the Earth. And yet the problem and solution are the same. The Earth, too, is in the same sort of wobble, because collectively humanity isn't balanced over its center, either.

To understand the wobble of our lives requires undressing the philosophy to which we've ascribed, going back to basics, and building a philosophy that reflects a process of inner growth. This requires searching with new eyes and with greater perception to discover the essential parts of our wellness. We've built a life philosophy that is no longer serving us, and so we are faced with venturing into new arenas to find and re-establish our inner balance.

## Embracing a New Philosophy for Living

Often, our philosophy for living doesn't extend into the spiritual dimension at all. We are involved mostly with solving our daily concerns, and these are focused on the tangible world of families, jobs, and lifestyles. We may be uncomfortable with words like *God*, *spirit*, and *soul*, or with the idea of adopting a spiritual philosophy for living, because in the past we haven't had to pay much attention to our spiritual lives.

A friend was telling me recently that her teenage son, who was in a drug rehabilitation center, was voicing a similar concern. She said that he was making progress reclaiming his emotions and accepting responsibility for his actions, but his stumbling block was the difficulty he had in figuring out what it meant when he was told to "turn his problem and the solution over to a Higher Power." He had no idea where to begin to find this Higher Power or even what It was.

If the truth were known, most people aren't very clear about what they believe. Yet when we are in spiritual crisis we are called upon to clarify our beliefs in order to identify our relationship with a Higher Power. We are part of a larger system of life in ways that we can see physically and in ways that we can perceive only intuitively. We have a physical relationship with the Earth, and the Earth in turn has an actual relationship with the Milky Way solar system, which is part of our galaxy and the universe. We are also bonded to these other living systems through an invisible sense, an energy, that is the basis of all life.

In order to heal through spiritual crisis we must learn that the tangible physical world is only the end result, not the place of beginnings. Energy comes before matter or the manifestation of matter. This means that the energy in our bodies or in the Earth's environment is influenced most radically by what we can't even see with our eyes. The harmony of energies of our bodies, minds, feelings, and spirits creates our health. A lack of spiritual energy in our lives or our bodies causes breakdown and eventual collapse just as it does within the sphere of any living thing.

## The Breath of Life: Life-force Energy

Ancient wisdom recognized energy as the basis for all life. Today, modern physics has created the bridge to join modern science with the wisdom of ancient cultures. In describing matter, physics has abandoned the old favorite, particle theory, in favor of unified field theory, in which matter is seen as energy. Energy is now accepted as the invisible life force maintaining all matter. The vocabulary is different for scientists and for sages, but the meaning is the same.

Life-force energy has for centuries been identified as "chi," the current of power surging through humans and nature, and as "prana," the Sanskrit term for energy, called the breath of life. Many cultures use the idea of energy to designate this invisible living essence that maintains our

well-being and that of all other living things. This subtle
energy flow is created and maintained by our emotional
well-being, our physical health, and our spiritual effort.
Energy isn't something we can observe with the naked
eye. Rather than seeing energy itself, we see the results of
different kinds of energy at work in our lives. We see
microwave ovens cooking our food, we know radio waves
bring us sound, we understand that the sun's rays give us
solar heat. Positive life-force energy keeps us alive and in
balance. When we are in need of healing or regaining our
emotional well-being, we can feel the ebb and flow of energy as we gain or lose health, gain or lose emotional assurance of our well-being, gain or lose the certainty of our participation with a loving God-force.

Years ago when I began to learn about spiritual energy
and to use this energy in healing, I discovered for myself
that this invisible and potent force that I felt in my hands or
sensed with my intuition was the basis for true healing and
the means through which people could help each other and
all living things. This life-force energy can actually be seen
around the human body through the special light-sensitive
photography known as Kirlian photography. What we all
need to know in order to heal is what creates and encourages energy and what decimates it.

## Spiritual Energy and a New Understanding of Love

When we are in spiritual crisis we find ourselves between
two worlds. One world is closing down; we can feel this in
our bodies when we are debilitated or in serious straits. We
can also observe this closing-down in our lifestyles because
we may for the first time be facing life as a single person, or
we may have lost some aspect of our familiar support struc-

ture or the hope of ever having a certain kind of life. Whatever the circumstances, we are painfully aware that the old lifestyle we've lived is disintegrating or has disintegrated.

As we watch our old, familiar lives falling away we sometimes assume the change means we may actually die. While that may sometimes be true, it doesn't need to be. The energy from our former lives has certainly left or is leaving. And to go forward with living we must identify our processes of change accurately and learn the ways of this newly-emerging energy of Love that is awakening within us. We feel newly-forming energy in, for example, the desire to find meaning in our lives, to offer something of value to others, and to find relationships that fill our deep inner emptiness and offer us unconditional Love and nurturing.

Trudy was a dancer, and her work was the way she shared her Love with others. For many years she had been sick, going from one medical center to another searching for a cause that no one could ever identify. She had always loved to dance and had, in fact, been trained as a ballerina at one of the finest schools. When her ten-year marriage collapsed, it seemed her illness would take over her life, and her future was almost being negated by her struggle. Then she began, after many years, to dance again. She found the Divine in the joy of dancing, and she dedicated her work to whatever service she might give through her art. This was Trudy's way of working through spiritual crisis. Taking one day at a time and letting her love of dance be her inspiration, she began to perform her own choreographed pieces, and slowly she emerged through disease and loss to inner peace and a meaningful life.

A new stream of energy pours into our lives and into the invisible energy environment of the Earth from the Universal Source of life-force energy. That is why most people feel the sting of loss in spiritual crisis at the same time they feel a fresh new impulse.  To understand the way this new energy affects our lives, we can think about turning on our television sets.  If we tune into a station that has already signed off the air, we get only static.  If we don't know that this station has signed off, then we miss the other shows that are coming in bright and clear on other channels.  We may wait for the static to clear.  We may bang the TV, rotate the dial or antenna frantically, or call the repair company and complain.  But when the broadcast beam has been discontinued at the station, nothing helps.

As we enter the twenty-first century a new spiritual broadcast beam is replacing the others.  If we are going to respond to this differently-focused energy, we will need to learn its characteristics and the ways to receive it in our lives and on the Earth.  This new energy is spiritual energy.  It's based on a fresh understanding of Love that incorporates both our relationship to our own inner truth and to the God-force system that includes all life.

I've come to see Love as the opportunity for all things to grow into their greatest potential while maintaining the balance of the whole.  Love as the opportunity of growth through balance is the major premise around which this book has been written, because Love is the organizing principle of holism and the holographic model after which our bodies and the universe are fashioned.

## Your Body and Your Life Are Meant to Be in Balance

A major way we can identify this emerging spiritual impulse in our lives is through our search for balance.  In order for our lives to be in balance, all its parts must be in harmony.  This means we must be in balance with those around us.

The people in this larger group or community must be in balance with ever-widening groups until all of humanity is touched. Humanity must then find balance with the Earth's living systems, and these with the solar system—and so on until the largest universal system is reached. Balance is therefore essential on the level of physical matter as well as in spiritual energy. Each aspect of energy, no matter how large, is built on the health and balance of the smallest of its parts. In the new science called Chaos Theory, this phenomenon is called the Butterfly Effect. It's defined as a "sensitive dependence on initial conditions," and it means that even the tiniest variable has an effect on results.[1]

The point is that your own balance or imbalance affects the entire God-force. No doubt you've heard the expression that when a child smiles, the energy of the farthest star is shifted.

A way to think about these complex interrelationships of the smallest to the largest entity is through the model of a hologram. A hologram is a three-dimensional photograph recorded on film by a reflected laser beam of a subject. Depending on the way you look at a hologram, you see a particular range of relationships of the individual elements. The picture you observe looks different from each perspective, and yet all aspects of the image are contained within the single picture. Apply this concept to your body, and you see quickly that what you observe as one surface is actually many planes that can be considered separately. The God-source level of life, spiritual energy, is the same, except that the holographic image is invisible. We experience spiritual energy through our evaluation of a situation once we are aware that the God-source influences are changing our lives.

The inclusive system of human being, humanity, Earth,

living things, all the way to the universe is a hologram, and
so is each of the individual parts. Our solar system is its
own hologram; so is the Earth, humanity, and the individual. We find holograms when we go inside the physical
body, too. A cell is a hologram, and even within a cell at
the nucleus we find visible and invisible components to the
holographic images of a complete and balanced living entity. This means that if we understand the ways in which
balance can be achieved among body, mind, and spirit,
then we can see the ways in which the largest system
works. Conversely, once we understand the ways in which
the macro systems work, we can determine the quality of
our own life's balances.

## Why Our Culture Is Breaking Down

Because the world is imbalanced, our physical, social, political, legal, medical, and religious systems are cracking apart
under the pressure of spiritual crisis. The spin-offs from
these breakdowns come in the guise of AIDS and other
immune-deficiency diseases; cancer that will shortly affect
one out of every two people; world-wide terrorism and
racial tension; banking corruption; millions of people
unable to afford health-care insurance; massive unemployment and shaky world economies; unimaginable starvation
and deprivation; and a dim future for the majority of children in the world.

As a culture, we find ourselves overwhelmed with people's needs and less and less able to provide the means to
stabilize either their bodies, their communities, or the social
and political agencies that we used to call on for help. We
and our society are in spiritual crisis. Rather than working
with the energy of the newly-emerging spiritual impulse,

the energy of holism, we are working against it. Any effort to heal our lives or our planet without acknowledging this spiritual impulse is like trying to swim upstream against a raging current.

## What Is Behind Loss and Disease?

We human beings are at a place in our evolutionary climb where anything can happen. We are at the boiling point, the point at which elements change form. Without doubt, we need courage, tenacity, and the desire for a different future to fuel our efforts in acknowledging this newly-emerging spiritual impulse. Likewise, in our own lives, when we face a life-threatening illness or loss of a loved one, a divorce, or a child with AIDS, we will need to draw loving energy from every hopeful thought, inspiration, prayer, or profound belief that we can muster. I once heard a Viet Nam veteran repeat the adage that there are no atheists in foxholes. Well, we are in our own foxhole in spiritual crisis, and it's time to get serious about what we really believe. Healing comes from genuine change rather than from crisis medicine. Change takes time, and we have no time to waste.

Unfortunately, we have developed the habit of looking squarely into the face of change only when we must. Because the personal experience of disease or loss brings home our own mortality so clearly, we try to look the other way as long as we can, and when we can no longer avoid confrontation with God, we finally ask what a dying woman wrote in her diary, "Why me, why now, why didn't I realize?"

Our intuitions alert us to what is really going on inside us and on the planet. When we say "I think," we mean something quite different from what we mean when we say

"I believe." When a thought is only a thought and never moves out of the rational stage, we can dismiss it without concern. But when a thought becomes a belief and we fail to honor this belief, we know in our hearts that there will be consequences. These consequences don't come from a vengeful God or a random one, either. They come as the natural result of cause and effect. When we operate in any particular way, our bodies, our thoughts and emotions, our intentions and actions, reap the return of what we've put out. We can observe from the returns on our current efforts that we must change our initiatives.

The way out of disease and loss comes from emulating an effectively functioning living system's modus operandi. What does this mean physically for healing? Because our bodies are connected to our minds, emotions, and spirits, and these are also interconnected with all their counterparts in every other living thing on the planet and beyond, it means that all elements nurture and sustain each other. Where one aspect is impaired, therefore, the entire system suffers. So when we awaken Love in our souls, we heal our lives. And when we heal our lives, we contribute to healing the Earth and the larger systems beyond.

## Stepping Out of Crisis and Toward Spiritual Wisdom

In working with small healing groups, I like to start our time together with questions that help uncover feelings we may never before have expressed in a group or even to ourselves. I recently asked a group of four women, "What is the most important quality your life lacks, the quality you want to claim for your future?" An insightful answer came from a slender, middle-aged woman who began by saying that she had for more than six years been undergoing various treatments for cancer. She said, "I want to set my spirit free and to find joy in my life. I want to do the things that up to this point I haven't dared to do, enjoy the experiences and adventures I've previously denied myself or felt I wasn't qualified for or good enough to deserve." She poured out her feelings as if she had never before realized these yearnings.

We find each productive step of our journey out of crisis by honoring the feelings that lie in the deepest, most immediately unreachable, part of our lives and our hearts. These are more than passing moods; rather, they are the emotional and spiritual framework of our lives needing acknowledgment. One of these significant emotional responses is joy, an intangible quality of appreciation for life that comes from our hearts—our spirits.

In order to move our journey along toward spiritual wisdom and subsequent health, we need to realize the ways in which our minds and our hearts function differently to maintain our physical and spiritual well-being. The heart connects the God-force with our own inner selves so that positive spiritual qualities can flow naturally into our lives. Our rational minds tell us whether or not we have a right to experience these spiritual qualities, like joy, which are emotions that generate substantial life-force energy for healing. Others are hope, compassion, trust, faith, and Love.

You may not know that you are looking for these qualities. In fact, you may be afraid to believe in a relationship with a benevolent Divine force because the pervasive misery on the Earth suggests that there is no God, or certainly not one who is powerful or caring. I choose rather to believe that this benevolent force hurts when we do, and although we live in accordance with the laws of this Earth, we are able through Love to invoke a new level of interaction and healing for all humanity.

When you place your belief in a Higher Power or God-force that is at the center of your life, you gain an immediate edge in healing. The treatments you undertake will be enhanced because you will be drawing serenity and healing potential from the God-source. Our individual healing efforts operate like the force of a single battery: when we plug ourselves into the generator of the God-force, our inner energy balance actually changes. While many remedies alleviate painful symptoms of disorders, in order to heal we need to find the more pervasive spiritual energy imbalances and root them out.

Your healing begins by trusting the process of spiritual change that has guided people's lives since earliest recorded history. Your future is meant to be filled with Love and community, even though you don't see it or can't even imagine it. You will find the guidance, support, and direct relationship with the God-source as you need it and cultivate it. The people who are to be involved in your life will find you as you seek to heal and recover if you simply allow a place for them in your life.

## Traditional Spiritual Crisis

As early as the twelfth century John-of-the-Cross first described the dark night of the soul and the surrender of one's spirit to a single divine authority. The steps in the traditional path of spiritual transformation began with the loss of meaning and purpose in life, then moved on to the struggle of abandonment, which was more than physical loss but a deeply poignant fear of being deserted by God or banished from God's presence. This was followed by a period of search for God in which one encountered one's own false gods, who tried to claim one's allegiance. And finally came the battle of the personal versus the Divine will, which ended in the release and metaphoric resurrection of the seeker.

This path toward God inevitably meant crossing the lowest and most fearsome inner passages: the place of utter desolation and abandonment, the dark night of the soul. Taking these steps meant that when one finally arrived at the other side of the spiritual quest, resurrection, one had achieved complete abandonment of the personal self. Spiritual crisis was, and is, an encounter with spiritual authority. As in a power play between two strong individuals, when one enters into spiritual crisis one engages in a power play with God in which the object is the release of one's personal will unto the will of the heavens—complete abandonment of the personal self.

## Contemporary Spiritual Crisis

We expect people who live a monastic life devoted to service to God to undergo such spiritual struggle as I have just described. But today we are being shown through the experience of crisis that we, too, are subject to spiritual law. We live in a time when we are being taught through spiritual crisis to value the basic spiritual principles upon which the entire universe functions. These spiritual truths are emerging from deep within our personal lives and our culture to re-affirm our connection to a God-force and to re-establish our lifeline of vital life-force energy in order to heal our lives and our Earth. No longer for the secular few, spiritual crisis is now a world-wide and fully planetary epidemic.

In this crisis, we are responsible for carrying our own weight and our part of the spiritual pact of living. We are undoubtedly being given the spiritual understanding to work with the Universe. Now, through the severity of spiritual crisis, our lives are exposed to experiences that both humble and inspire us and certainly teach us that we are but an aspect of a mysterious greater whole.

Medical intuitive and healer Caroline Myss talks about this change in relationship to God by suggesting that we are emerging from our parent-child relationship with God, a relationship in which we expected to be fed, clothed, and provided for. The changing spiritual energy of our time, she suggests, is birthing a different and co-creative relationship with the God-force.[2]

Spiritual crisis is our present-day spiritual gauntlet even though we may or may not have a meaningful relationship with God through organized religion. We are spiritual beings living on a sentient planet, and so eventually and inevitably we will need to come to this recognition. Spirituality professes no single set of convictions but is rather an all-inclusive path toward service to the God-force. This newly emerging spiritual path is opening up to every individual because the Sacred lives and is expressed through ordinary actions within each of our lives.

## Walking a Razor's Edge—Seeking Balance

Our lives have a purpose regardless of what we may think now. Sometimes the humbling process of getting seriously ill, or losing everything, or seemingly needing to start all over again forces us to direct our lives in a new, healthier, more balanced direction. The effect of this humbling process might be what we would call "Universal Tough Love."

Your journey through spiritual crisis has its own energy and time line specific to your personal spiritual learning curve. You are in transformation, and the days ahead will take form only one day at a time. You and the energy of the God-source are designing your future according to the principles of balance and holism and your newly-emerging spiritual partnership. The old is being pulled out of your grasp. A meditation card from the *The Course in Miracles* says it well: "All your past except its beauty is gone, and nothing is left but a blessing."[3]

Our responsibility is to build on that blessing, to identify what we do know that is positive about our lives and to grow from that place. From the accumulating tension and ferocious trauma in our lives we are being directed to look toward our own inner wisdom. We are being pushed toward a view of life that is holistic and life-revering, one that offers renewed hope, creativity, and inspiration for facilitating positive change.

In life we must try to achieve balance: a balance among our inner energies, a balance between our inner, meditative, spiritual world and our outer, physical, workaday world, a balance between our needs and our wants, between our intentions and our actions. Living in ways that produce inner satisfaction and joy is achieved through balance, and so healing is also achieved through balance. Balance is a key to successful healing because it draws us back toward our own centers. Because we've been living out of balance for so long, we may not recognize our true centers when we've found them. The abnormal at first feels more like the normal. Healing involves shifting this perception to where we are aware of our center and can adjust our lives accordingly.

Balancing the parts of our lives means balancing energy. As the basic building block of all matter, energy is the subtlest form of creation, yet the most enduring. Thoughts, feelings, and spiritual energy are real, and their effect is tangible in our bodies. Old habits are difficult to break and to replace with new ways of thinking about our lives and our health. Keeping the discipline of a newly-initiated course of endeavor is like walking a razor's edge: we keep falling off. When we do fall off, part of the spiritual journey is keeping the balance between self-acceptance of our human limitations at the time and self-generated reassurance that we are capable of beginning again. We know we're making substantial progress when we accept this pattern as normal and we no longer even take note of our failure, only of our persistence and dedication to a continuing effort. When our self-deprecating talk stops, our concentration on the daily doing begins in earnest. The act of searching for the Sacred becomes fulfillment enough.

## Honoring the Personal Passage on the Spiritual Trail

As we heal we find many people in our lives who need help and whom we want to help. Often, we are so convinced of the truth of our way that we may overpower others with our well-intentioned ideas and initiatives. When people are in severe pain or greatly distressed from loss, they feel without roots—totally lost. They want an instant philosophy that will help and are inclined quite naturally to be persuaded easily. Yet if you've ever noticed the teaching styles of those teachers you enjoyed and learned the most from, you'll recall that you learned effortlessly from them. We naturally want to discover our relationship with our world, and this doesn't stop when we turn three, or ten, or fifty-five, or eighty-two years old. I've found that time on the spiritual trail makes all of us less certain about everything save the moment and the truth of the God-force as we perceive it. In the long run, experience is always the best teacher anyway, because we trust most completely what we've experienced personally rather than what others have told us.

The journey on which we have embarked through spiritual crisis requires that we come to honor our passage as the sacred transformation that it is. Divine authority, the Loving Source of all creation, can become as familiar to us as the faces of our children or partners and as intriguingly different as each evening's sunset. Expecting the unexpected, living with questions, searching for and finding approval from yourself, finding balance and center for the first time— these are all part of the spiritual adventure you have undertaken. Expect that you are in for the journey of your life.

## NOTES

1. James Gleick, *Chaos, Making a New Science* (New York, NH: Viking Penguin, 1987), p.23.

2. Caroline Myss, "Healing Our Wounds," *Convergence Magazine* (Concord, NH:  1991).

3. Helen Schuckman, *The Course in Miracles* (Huntington Station, NY:  Foundation for Inner Peace, 1980).

# 2 Major Physical and Emotional Loss Leads to Spiritual Insights

*The hand of the Divine awakens you to the inevibility of life change.*

When we are in pain, we know our bodies are hurting in some way. When we've been rejected or reviled by someone, we readily accept and acknowledge the emotions that flood forth immediately. In spiritual crisis, while physical and emotional factors are in play, it is our spirits that are hurting—crimped and confined and cut off from influencing our lives. Our physical complaints and emotional responses are easy to identify. What are the symptoms when our spirits are hurting? They are the symptoms caused by our desire for Love.

Spiritual energy is Love. And Love is our opportunity to grow into the fullest expression of ourselves while maintaining the balance of the whole. This means that Love is the encouraging energy of our lives, the part that pushes us forward when we want to hang back, tells us we can be successful when the world tells us we cannot. Love awakens us to our true depth and exquisite nature and to our enduring connection to God.

When we are totally preoccupied with our lives, we feel less certain about who we are and what we are trying to accomplish. We feel less in touch with our natural creativity, intuition, and the part of ourselves that is whole and beautiful. These are the symptoms of a sick spirit. When we are cut off from Love, we are cut off from the transcendent quality of our humanness. We become the least we can be rather than the most, and we lose our capacity to expect great and generous actions and initiatives from ourselves and others.

The more distress we're in at present, the less inner quiet space we seem to have available to us to free up this Love. Trying to meditate or even analyze our emotional or spiritual beliefs is a hundred times more difficult when we are in the depths of trauma. And yet this is the dilemma many of us now face. As when we fail to practice preventive medicine, we tend to take the vitamins after we're already sick. Perhaps it's human nature to wait until we're in a crisis to ask the basic questions.

## Spiritual Crisis: An Issue of Love and Relationships

In healing we are challenged to help our bodies and to learn a positive approach to our life problems, but there is more. We are searching for the transcendent quality that lifts us beyond our limitations into our expansiveness. This transcendent quality is, in fact, Love, and yet this ebullient energy comes from humble beginnings. We find Love by identifying our spiritual imbalances. The word "imbalance" seems like such an unassuming and innocuous word to be at the root of the most grievous struggles of our lives. Yet we know that a seed always precedes the tree and that an idea comes before the full-blown initiative. So it is not unrealistic to accept that the largest, most dismal experiences in which we may be living began as basic spiritual imbalances.

We think of spiritual crisis as a breakdown of sorts. Actually, spiritual crisis is a break-through to the reservoir of Love, spiritual energy, held captive within us and replaceable from the God-source. When we tap this reservoir we are able to give ourselves the Love that is essential for life. We tend to think of Love as an emotion rather than a spiritual energy, and so we consider it extraneous: nice if you have it but acceptable if you don't. That isn't true, because Love is the regulator of our living environments. The energy of spiritual Love creates and maintains the quality of our physical and emotional environments.

In spiritual crisis it is our living environments that are altered. Sometimes this means the physical environment of our bodies; other times it means the emotional environment of our relationships with partners, children, extended family, and working colleagues. When we seek healing and forward momentum toward a meaningful life, we must consider the ways we presently use Love and our effectiveness in internalizing its energy.

When we are immersed in hopelessness or anxiety, we aren't interested in benefits to be derived at some future date. We are shocked and fractured on a level often so deep that we feel as if we may be sucked down a deep drain. This is not the time to be rational about our spirituality but one in which we need to begin to live with a prayer in our hearts, a prayer that offers us Love from this larger system, the God-source. A client of mine expressed this feeling as "being remembered by God and accepting that healing is taking place even though I am too preoccupied and drawn inside to apply any mental effort to facilitate this process."

Life in spiritual crisis is like a Zen *koan*. A *koan* is a cosmic puzzle of sorts that Japanese Zen masters give their students to meditate upon. These thoughts are meant to stop the mind's activity and turn the awareness inward. In other words, you can't figure it out, you can only accept it, in terms that force you to transcend self-induced limitations. "What is the sound of one hand clapping?" is an example. Acceptance is exactly what you need in spiritual crisis—not a search for rational explanations but an acceptance that you are in a cosmic puzzle that defies your immediate understanding because you are meant to go inside and transcend your own self-defining limitations.

## People Who Are Healing—Case Examples

In the course of my work with clients, I've identified four types of physical disruption that alter the status quo of our most familiar and trusted living environments. These four alterations seem to bring on what I'm defining as spiritual crisis: a breakdown in our relationship with our own whole-ness and with the God-force. All of these breakdowns or break-throughs deal with the quality of the Love we receive and the ways in which we allow this Love to nurture us deeply. The four types of physical disruption and the way they manifest themselves are listed below, beginning with the environment in which the disruption occurs and ending with the way we experience that kind of disruption.

1. *Living environment:*      One's physical body
   *Identified through:*      Severe, recurring, or life-threatening illness

2. *Living environment:*      One's family unit
   *Identified through:*      Breakdown or loss of an essential family bond

3. *Living environment:*      One's job and partnership
   *Identified through:*      Repeated failure in career and/or partnerships

4. *Living environment:*      One's lifestyle
   *Identified through:*      Dramatic and compressed change altering one's lifestyle

These four physical disruptions spur us to try to heal our losses, not with an eye to pretending that the circumstances never happened but with a sense that all things have led to our greater learning and that balancing our lives and our world is primarily our responsibility, in partnership with the Universe.

Not everyone who wants to heal does heal. Other unfathomable factors intercede to bring us face to face with a vast God-space that we don't control. But everyone who tries is helped; everyone who searches sincerely finds a measure of relief and comfort. We can add to and subtract from many aspects of our healing or recovery programs, but in order to heal we must have a sense of the way we fit with a larger, all-encompassing life-force. Sometimes people are more comfortable calling God by other names. For many, the term "God" brings to mind an anthropomorphic image of a man-made deity. The God-system we are discussing in this book is God as energy: an expansive force that is outside human design and yet available to us in ways that are both personal and specific.

I've found in my work with clients that conversations taking us beyond the rational and into the experiential realms of spirituality are the most satisfying. People want to feel God's presence even more than they want to know God intellectually.

## Pain Plays a Part in Your Life Dramas

In our search to know God, we encounter different types of pain that inevitably play a part in our life dramas. We each handle pain differently. Some repress it, others feel awash in uncontrollable emotions, some tough it out, and others accept it as if it were the inevitable consequence of life. The rare person can acknowledge the pain and at the same time move inward, seeking a new interpretation for his or her life and for the challenge being faced. Most people aren't afraid to die, they are afraid they will be a burden to their families, or they are afraid that they may be in unmanageable pain at the end. When we can even dare to consider that a gift lies beneath such struggle, we pull the barb from our hearts. If we can find a reason for it all, even a shred of understanding that tells us something good can come from our pain, we can accept it. Many people are shocked to realize that they do have options, that they can prolong the quality of their lives more than anticipated, and that they can also heal in ways that have little to do with the physical medicines they take. Our spirits are capable of wielding the sort of Love energy that heals when we accept an active relationship with the God-source.

# Healing Observations from Those Experiencing Severe, Recurring, or Life-threatening Illness

When we get sick and stay sick we often feel as if our bodies have failed us. After all, this is the body that we've trusted, the one we've tried to take care of, the one that has seen us through many years and experiences. How could this be happening? How can we get at this disease or breakdown, this invisible assailant that is robbing us of our future?

We must first understand that the enemy is imbalance rather than disease, which is only the symptom. The antidote to disease always involves opening our hearts, taking the barricades down from around our spirits, and accepting our lives and ourselves in ways that are new to us. Such release frees up spiritual energy to help us heal our physical bodies and ignite a future we have yet to claim.

## *Sue, Molly, and John Experienced the Breakdown of Their Physical Bodies through Life-threatening Disease.*

*Sue* has two children and three grandchildren. She lives alone in a small, attractive apartment. Sue has an inoperable tumor.

Confronting our own death is the single biggest issue any of us will ever face. No struggle on any of our horizons looms larger than this consideration. And at the same time no consideration is any more freeing than the realization that we can leave this Earth if we've been miserable. We usually assume that sick people want to heal so that they can return to the lives they've lived, but often this isn't the case. Sue, like many, wants to stay on the Earth only if she can find a reason worth healing for, a way to be of value. Although she's had a wide variety of jobs, they've all fallen short of the inner mark. She recognizes that she's been a person who has "lived in her head," and thus her challenge in healing is to open her heart to finding the Love that can set her free, either in this world or the next.

Sue is an extraordinary woman, and after spending time working with her I often wonder who the client is. Her search is the classic struggle of spiritual crisis through the dark night of the soul. Her deepest longing is to feel the presence of the God-force in her life and to accept unequivocally this bonded relationship that will carry her soul through all eternity. She recognizes that the effort to heal is enormous, and her desire to heal must carry equal weight.

*A MEANINGFUL SPIRITUAL TRUTH: Healing changes from a possibility to a probability when you experience a relationship with the God-force. Healing happens every minute of every day when you are open to seeing what you've never seen before. Tomorrow has not yet been written—you and God are writing it now.*

*Molly* is a middle-aged wife and mother. She is happily married and has four small children. She wasn't surprised when she was diagnosed with cancer. She made some important changes in her life before the subsequent surgery and felt she had finished with cancer, but several years later the cancer reappeared. This time she delved deeper into the emotions that had set her up for disease. She attended workshops and lectures and tried to integrate what she'd learned. Molly was operated on a second time and again felt she had finished with cancer. A year and a half later the cancer reappeared. Her response was extremely telling:

she said that she knew she still had not connected with that inner place that would keep her on the Earth. She went on to tell me that a certain state of mind and heart existed when she thought she might die: a pressing attention to the present moment. After each surgery, when she assumed she would be fine, that pressing attention to inner balance dissipated. She felt this time she knew the feeling that she was after, and she vowed she would never again lose it.

*A MEANINGFUL SPIRITUAL TRUTH: Healing means that an inner spiritual imbalance has been corrected. These imbalances are observed only through your inner senses and God's Grace. If you were not surprised to get sick, you should not be surprised to heal.*

*John* was fifty-four when he had a massive heart attack. During the attempts to resuscitate him, his heart stopped, and for a short period of time he was legally dead. He later recounted the entire procedure to his surgeon, having observed it from above the operating table. He felt that his life had changed irrevocably because he realized that death was not the end of consciousness.

While observing his body, he said, he met an angel, a spiritual teacher, who told him to go back, that he had important healing work to do. I met John after this experience because he felt that the spiritual teacher he had met in his out-of-body experience was, in fact, the spiritual energy that I'd written about as initiating my own spiritual journey many years previously.

Out-of-body experiences are no longer unusual, with more than ten million Americans claiming to have such experiences every year.[1] Such experiences affirm for people that their lives have specific significance and often head them back into physical reality with renewed energy and certainly a sense of purpose. Once we have verified to our own satisfaction that the spiritual realm is real, then we can move on to learning to use spiritual energy in everyday life in meaningful ways.

*A MEANINGFUL SPIRITUAL TRUTH: A blessing comes from the spiritual realm to confirm that you matter and that your life has significance. When you accept a blessing, you invite the God-source to teach and enlighten you in all that you do.*

## Healing Observations from Those Experiencing Breakdown or Loss of Essential Family Bonds

Propagation is the way the world stays peopled and filled with living things. When we form bonds with partners and children, we are forming intimate and lasting energy dynamics that affect most directly our physical health and well-being. Making love is of course more than a sexual act, it is a decidedly spiritual one. When we honor this belief whether or not the relationship lasts, both people have benefited from the experience. When making love is devoid of spiritual energy, both people lose energy. This means that the circulatory and reproductive systems are weakened by repeatedly sleeping with people with whom no mutual spiritual growth is experienced.

The relationship between spirituality and the immune system is extremely significant. We see the vast numbers of people getting sick with these disorders, and we think these diseases come from viruses that we must track down and from global pollutants and contaminants. Certainly, there are viruses and staggering poisons in our atmosphere and ground, but we are susceptible to these diseases to the degree that we are devoid of active spiritual energy supporting our immune systems. As spiritual crisis awakens the spiritual impulse on our planet, the God-source is also awakening our personal spiritual energy and requiring us to enhance or discover the spiritual components in all our relationships.

## *Joan and Brad Encountered Spiritual Crisis through a Breakdown of an Essential Family Bond.*

*Joan* called me because she couldn't seem to get her life tracked again after losing her son to AIDS. In addition, an x-ray of her lung showed a shadow the size of a grapefruit. It seems that when we lose children or partners to immune-deficiency diseases, we are being told that issues of personal co-creation with the God-force are at stake. Our physical health—specifically, our immune systems—may be at risk unless we are able to restore spiritual love to our lives.

Joan had been married for many years and described her relationship as "satisfactory, neither positive nor negative, just a fact of life." She did have strong feelings for the son she'd lost, however, and felt bitter and guilty that he'd died so young. At his death he was only twenty-six. Joan naturally expected she would have years to be with her son, and so she acquiesced to his wish to move west for "just a few years." He never returned but died soon after being diagnosed with AIDS. She felt rejected by life, filled with rage at those who had spurned her son because of the nature of his disease. She was deeply lost in an effort to understand why God had allowed this to happen.

When we lose a child, no matter at what age, a part of

the established pattern of our energy field now has no place to go. The person we have loved is no longer available to us to love. What do we do with this Love? It's like putting on a coat with only one pocket: what do we do with the other hand on a cold, blustery day?

Energy patterns are formed through Love, and when we lose the person we were bonded to, the Love needs to be drawn back into our spiritual selves rather than immediately reinvested in another person. Author Regina Ryan, in her book *No Child in My Life*,[2] identifies this spiritual energy as "wise innocence," or the return to our basic God-qualities but with a present sense of maturity and wisdom.

True and lasting spiritual insight and growth comes from our willingness to draw the pain of loss back into our hearts and our physical bodies, thereby honoring the cycles of life that do often include loss and transition. This energy of Love for another nurtures us in everlasting ways and expands our capacity to love again with renewed strength and vigor. In some sense the Love we've shared with the person we've lost is the seed, the impulse, that will eventually go out from our hearts to another. Even if our relationships have strong overtones of pain, trauma, guilt, frustration, betrayal, or grief, we are nevertheless required to reclaim the Love from the bond and relinquish the rest.

*A MEANINGFUL SPIRITUAL TRUTH: Healing the heart means healing your soul. But since your soul is already whole, then healing comes through listening to your soul's wisdom and accepting new ways to recapture the Love you need.*

*Brad's* wife was dead after many long years of being in a nursing home. She had died of Alzheimer's Syndrome. Brad was a friend of the family, and so our time together was more of a sharing between friends than a counseling session. I was told by a family member that he needed help in getting on with his life because he still seemed so lost without his partner of many years. In our conversation, Brad wanted only to talk about his wife in the most glowing terms: their relationship and history together for the thirty-five years they had been married. He spoke of his own life in an offhand way, as if what he did really didn't matter much, implying that he was perfectly happy living with his memories. Can we have a meaningful life sustained only by our memories?

Like Brad, we may be in spiritual crisis and yet be unable to recognize that we are, because the circumstances seem normal and our responses justified and appropriate. When we lose someone we love, we are supposed to grieve. When we get divorced or separated we are handed an entirely different set of emotions that we are told are appropriate. Memories hold energy charges, and replaying these memories incessantly becomes an addiction. Yet each time we pull up a highly-charged memory, we feel less and less of that charge. When our life's purpose becomes only to support our past memories, we move from circumstances that are normal in loss to those that are a hidden form of spiritual crisis. When a memory wants to fade and we refuse to let it, we are supporting it with our own life-force energy. This drains us physically and emotionally and keeps us from having any sort of present-life involvement.

*A MEANINGFUL SPIRITUAL TRUTH: Physical and emotional healing is necessary only for those still in physical life. You heal as you accept the challenge of the present and allow the energy from your past to fade. Those you've loved and lost remain part of your loving energy. Your challenge is to accept the experience as your gift and go on.*

## Healing Observations from Those Experiencing Repeated Failure in Career and/or Partnerships

We can always account for our failures through the inadequacies and ineptitudes of others. The first or second time a job or relationship doesn't work, we assume rightly that there may have been mitigating circumstances. Yet for many people, as they move through life, the string of failures mount. Eventually, hope is diminished, self-worth has long since been abandoned, and people are merely hanging onto the shadow of a meaningful life.

### Nancy and Greg Experienced Loss through Repeated Failure in Career and/or Partnerships.

Consider to what degree the "sins of the father" are passed to the son. Can we, or should we, blame our parents for the difficulties we encounter in our lives? Without doubt, we are marked irrevocably by our experiences as young, impressionable children. Yet certain children grow up in seriously dysfunctional households and remain unscathed while others in the same family develop serious pathologies and deeply-ingrained, self-defeating patterns of behavior. What makes the difference? It's our relationship to the Universe. That's because in addition to parental influence, another strategic influencing factor comes into play in our formative years: that of our relationship to the Universe and the reason we are on the Earth in the first place. What are we to learn in this lifetime? We need to learn of our spiritual paths and can do so by observing the patterns in our lives.

The patterns we experience are repetitive mini-life dramas that have something spiritual to teach us even though we may be unable to identify these patterns and their inherent issues at the time. Hindsight in spiritual work offers us good and valuable insights because we learn from our past and from reflecting on the patterns we now see. Often, when we consider the ways in which we've been the most jarred by life, we see that the feelings and beliefs associated with those traumas are the same each time. These issues and beliefs will keep returning in various forms all throughout our lives because they are keys we must use to unlock our spiritual paths. When we are able to identify these beliefs that are the steppingstones to spiritual wisdom, we can address our vulnerabilities before they again work their way into our physical lives.

*Greg* was voted by his high-school class the boy most likely to succeed. Yet Greg was in his fifties before he knew what success really meant. When a split separates our feelings from our intellect, we make the choices others want rather than the ones we need. Greg's story is not an uncommon one: many people feel they were influenced inappropriately to marry or not marry a certain person, to attend a certain college or any college at all, or to enter a particular field of study or career or not to do so. These same people later on in life often blame their parents, teachers, family, or others to whom they listened. People accept the influence of others because they trust other people's opinions more than they trust their own. In such cases the God-source is no doubt suggesting that we need to weigh our own intuitive wisdom most heavily.

Greg kicked around through many minimum-wage jobs until he accepted that he didn't know what he was doing, stopped battling the world, and began to accept that he had feelings that counted. At this point he found the difference between a job and meaningful work. He discovered that when you put your heart into work that springs from your own abilities and skill, in return you receive personal satisfaction, an increased belief in yourself and your capabilities, joy, feelings of self-worth, and the ability to also have a loving regard for other people and other living things.

*A MEANINGFUL SPIRITUAL TRUTH: Healing means working from your heart. And working means accepting that the ways you spend your time and effort not only contribute to your personal spiritual growth and satisfaction but also to the positive energy essential for global change.*

*Nancy* was so sweet it made your teeth hurt, as the saying goes. She was everyone's best friend, always available, always smiling, always everything everyone wanted. Nancy never talked about herself because she was too busy fixing everyone else. I met Nancy when she and her partner Joan came for counseling. It's easy to think that perhaps this all-giving and always-giving behavior and attitude means Love. Actually, this struggle to find ourselves comes from the deprivation of Love. We often love others as a substitute for loving ourselves, and so it is easier and more fulfilling to be in other people's shoes solving their problems. This is because our life issues seem too enormous to ever tackle.

Life in spiritual crisis keeps us within the energy of change by making readily accessible to us the spiritual lessons we are to engage. When we are in this particular pattern of "Repeated Failure in Career and/or Partnership," we find that all the people we love and those with whom we try to create lasting partnerships or career relationships fall away. We can't imagine what we are doing wrong, and for years we battle with the world we see rather than the one we feel or believe in.  Eventually, we realize that the problem lies not in what we are "doing," it's in what we are "being"— or, rather, not being:  ourselves.

Personal discovery was an enthralling experience for Nancy as she began to see what she was required to become—herself—and the challenge and lifelong process that this would be.  One of our most self-defeating ways of approaching any required change is to feel that we can accomplish it overnight.  When we set a date on our calendars and tell ourselves that we will be fixed by that time, of course we're setting ourselves up to fail.  Every significant change is a process, not a goal, and changing our expectations from the one to the other allows us to break the pattern of repeated failures.

Nancy has changed so dramatically—in her looks, her personality, her sense of herself—that no one would recognize her as the person she once was.  She has gone back to school and even to graduate school.  She is in another relationship that has lasted for a number of years.  She is her own person; calmness and a self-contained sense of purpose pervade her personality.  She knows she has broken the pattern of repeated failure, yet accepts that each day she will have additional inner work to do.

*A MEANINGFUL SPIRITUAL TRUTH:  Healing arises from the realization that each day is a fresh beginning requiring your attention to the spiritual teachings of that day.*

## Healing Observations from Those Experiencing Dramatic and Compressed Change

We can accept changes within our bodies more easily than changes that affect our family units or the lifestyle we've lived. I remember reading about the many people affected by the Great Depression of 1929 who, rather than face life without their accustomed lifestyles, jumped from high windows to their deaths. Beneath lifestyle issues are surely those of our own self-worth and even a sense of feeling safe in the world. We've been brought up to believe that if we work hard now, we will enjoy the fruits of our labor later on. When our lifestyles crash, we confront our beliefs in the Puritan work ethic that says, "But we gave up everything to create or have this future! How can this be happening? It isn't fair!" When our future is snatched from us, we feel as if life's safety net has suddenly evaporated and we are falling out of control through a dark and dangerous universe.

### Sophia and Elizabeth Experienced Dramatic and Compressed Change Altering their Lifestyles.

*Sophia* was unprepared for poverty. She and her husband both had reasonable educations, and yet within six months of each other they were laid off from their jobs. At first they assumed they would be able to get other work. But week after week produced nothing, and they gradually slid into hopelessness. Sophia recounts one of her lowest moments when she walked by a car that had a Garfield toy stuck on the back window. She remembers thinking what it would mean to her to have the fifteen dollars that had been spent on that toy: "I could buy a chicken for dinner, some potatoes, and broccoli. I could buy some apple juice for my two-year old. I could give my family something decent to eat."

Poverty diminishes our self-worth and our capacity to

expect Love.  Often, no Love is forthcoming from the agencies that are supposed to care, and most other people seem preoccupied and unaware of the desperate nature of our struggle.  We feel rejected by society, useless, and our lives become distended with fear.  Large-scale poverty is the symptom of a culture in spiritual crisis.  People, many thousands, even millions of people, drop continually through society's safety net.  Unless we individually make an effort to stem this freefall, much of the energy essential for planetary community will be lost.

Sophia was a good writer and, out of desperation, began to write about her family's plight.  Newspapers picked up the story, and soon caring messages, money, and job offers began to appear.  Sophia had reached out to tell the personal story of a family caught in the quicksand of poverty, and in helping herself she also awakened the energy of Love in the hearts of many others.

*A MEANINGFUL SPIRITUAL TRUTH: Healing requires you to sometimes be a pioneer by telling of the conditions that are prevalent and seriously destructive to human beings and human culture.  Through your efforts you awaken the Love within yourself and others.  This is the path toward global transformation.*

*Elizabeth* was in her mid-forties when she decided to leave her unhappy marriage and move far away from her parents, who made her feel guilty and inadequate.  She had for years imagined a time when she would, for once, have the courage to do something she wanted.  Intuitively, she knew she needed to live by herself for a period of time in order to heal.  She also realized that the thought terrified her.

I first met Elizabeth when she moved to New England. By the time I met her she was already comfortable talking about her need for spiritual growth and was quite easily able to assess her emotional "sinkholes" and what needed to be done to change old patterns. Elizabeth, like most of us, knew intellectually what she needed to do, but it is in the doing, day by day, that we change old patterns and allow our newly-balanced selves to emerge as the dominant force guiding our lives.

Strangely, one of Elizabeth's most profound experiences occurred when she was preparing to leave New England after a year. She recounts that she was driving off an exit ramp from a major interstate highway when she passed a woman driving toward her going the wrong way. She swerved out of the way, commenting out loud, "Look at that woman, she's going the wrong way and she doesn't even know it." She felt a strange twinge as she spoke these words but dismissed the incident, failing to see in it any relevance to her own life.

It is difficult to know when we are ready to relax our healing program a little and get on with normal living. Also important is recognizing what it means to relax our program without forgetting it totally. We alone are responsible for monitoring our imbalance as well as our healing progress. This subtle awareness is similar to what fishermen refer to as "keeping tension on the line." This means not too much slack and not too much play—just the right amount of pressure and effort produces the desired result.

One of the ways we monitor our lives spiritually is by paying attention to guidance coming through unlikely circumstances. What "messages" do we uncover in the normal course of a day that we dismiss and yet might be wise to take personally? Many months later, Elizabeth recalled the incident on the exit ramp and wished she had taken it more to heart as guidance for her own life.

A MEANINGFUL SPIRITUAL TRUTH: *Healing is effected in subtle as well as obvious ways. As we awaken inner Love, we expand our intuitive capacity. Expect that you will see and experience obvious and direct guidance for your life.*

## All Experiences, Large or Small!

Your past is behind you; even yesterday, as important as it felt, is only a fading energy. Today is your challenge, and tomorrow will take care of itself. Although you thought your crisis was limited to your health, your family, your partner, or your career or lifestyle, it is actually your spirit that needs attention. The energy in your life can be put to good use to create a desirable and meaningful future as you accept that your search for happiness and meaning has an essential spiritual aspect to it.

Our lives are like expensive cloisonne´ bowls that come by their beauty through the unique character of each individual piece. We are not works of art molded from one standard form. By the time we come to leave this earth, our lives should be a collection of individual experiences and expressions of ourselves and our Love. If they aren't, then we've missed the point of life. Like a horseback rider who is so timid she never risks any adventure for fear of falling off her horse, if we've never fallen, or failed, or risked, then we've never pushed our limits, and we have no idea of our ultimate potential. And for those people who feel they're risked yet never benefited, I offer the thought that the kind of risk we're talking about is the risk we take when we have nothing invested emotionally in either proving or disproving anything. This means we are open to learn from the risk-taking rather than just proving what we already believe.

Each of the four avenues of change we've discussed in this chapter lead to spiritual transformation. When we alter our perception we let in the goodness from others, the opportunities in life, the self-expression that encourages the development of our feeling of self-worth. All our experiences and all our memories and all our relationships are meant to build us as a spiritual energy-fortress. While we can and must lower the drawbridge for others and engage in meaningful relationships, nevertheless we—the spiritual energy of creation made manifest in physical form—stand alone against the winds and storms and attacking armies of life.

Spiritual crisis changes us, as it must to reach toward a future we little understand. Yet reaching, pushing, daring is what life is all about. Consider that:.

- life is a spiritual journey, and you are here for a reason.
- those who are in your life are meant to be there, whether they are playing a major role or a minor one, a positive or negative one.
- life has many unexpected turns that offer you unique and positive opportunities. Assume that change brings you life's best rather than its worst.


## NOTES

1. International Association for Near Death Studies, 638 Prospect Avenue, Hartford, CT 06105.

2. Regina Ryan, *No Child in my Life* (Walpole, NH: Stillpoint Publishing, *1993*).

# 3 Love and the Six Influences of Spiritual Energy

*Love is your opportunity to grow into the fullest expression of your potential while maintaining your balance within the whole.*

Love has been written about, sung about, considered, analyzed, and prayed over. You might think that with Love being the center of attention for so long, we would have figured out what it really is. Yet Love remains elusive.

We all know we should love each other and be caring and compassionate with all living things. And the golden rule has been around for a long time. Yet Love is more than an emotional response—although this is the guise in which we usually first discover it. Love is an energy, the most significant and essential energy of life. In this book, I've capitalized the "L" in the noun *Love* to suggest the potential we have when we consider Love, or loving each other, or the Earth, or the God-force.

Love as an energy supports our spiritual growth and forms the medium within which we as people can grow most successfully.

As we enter the twenty-first century, the energy of the God-force, Love, is assuming a more pressing and persistent influence in our lives. We are Love—and yet we don't know what that means. We are learning very slowly that it means we are invisible spiritual energy manifested in human form. We are just as real and just as much spiritual energy when we have moved beyond human form. Other living things are also just as much spiritual energy, although they have other physical presences than ours: animal, plant, tree, moon, star, universe. We human beings have bodies, and we have feelings, and we have the memory of our experiences and rational thought. Throughout our physical lives all of this grows together, inter-twined with our spiritual energy of Love, so that we are unable to single out any one part of our total "body-mind-spirit self" as separate from the rest.

The health of our physical bodies is based on the health and well-being of our emotions, which is in turn based on our exchange of Love with the Divine. We are being compelled through spiritual crisis to learn more about these spiritual natures of ours because we want to heal ourselves and our planet. To accomplish this requires our learning about Love as the basic energy of all life—the universal truth that is relevant for all living things wherever they live and whatever form they are in.

## Love as the Pervasive Energy of All Life

The energy of Love is universal and eternal. By that I mean that this energy never dies but is renewed each time it is used. Because Love is universal, its influence continually touches and nurtures all living things. The energy of Love is real: we can feel it when it is present, and we certainly feel its absence when we're living without it. Psychotherapist, scientist, and mystic Joan Borysenko in her extraordinary book, *Guilt is the Teacher, Love is the Lesson*, relates an experience from one of her clients who saw the energy of Love. The client explained, "I turned around and saw a ball of incredibly bright light hovering in the doorway. It was made out of—I don't know any other way to put this, but—well, love energy. There's no way to explain it really—you just know you're in the presence of God—held and loved."[1]

It is impossible to heal without using Love both for ourselves and for others. We are formed with this energy, and when we don't use it we are deviating from our natural design. We are learning about spiritual energy so that in our own way we can take the steps necessary to put this spiritual vigil first in our lives. What would it mean if we looked for Love in everyone as well as in ourselves? We'd see more Love and less anger and hate. We'd perpetuate the energy of healing everywhere we went and with every thought and action we experienced.

Healing on the physical level relieves pain; healing on the emotional level relieves stress from loss; and healing on the spiritual level produces the energy of Love so that it is the dominant influence in our bodies, minds, and lives. Spiritual healing is the basis of physical and emotional healing because it requires us to re-sort our entire way of functioning and thinking.

A spiritual search is a life search, and it is monitored not in the way we feel each day but in the overall quality and depth of our spiritual wisdom and insight gathered over a lifetime. If we could chart our spiritual growth, we'd see a slowly climbing line with many setbacks, some of them severe. These deep dips are the times we question everything about our foregone assumptions. These periods are throwbacks to our periods of greatest fear, when we felt isolated from the God-source.

In learning spiritually and accepting the ups and downs of this lifelong search, we come inevitably to the realization that we are made of the same "stuff," the very same energy of Love, as the Divine itself. We are made in the likeness of the God-force, and when we recognize this we become absorbed into Love and lose our fear. We may come to love ourselves by first loving God, or we may come to love God by first finding Love in ourselves; either way, we feel the power of Love. I'm reminded of the search Shirley MacLain chronicles in her book, *Out on a Limb*. As she begins her spiritual search she is unsure of her relationship with God and is told by a fellow spiritual seeker to stand on the beach and repeat, "I am God." At first she finds this extremely difficult. Her response reflects the feeling most of us begin with, that we are separate from the Divine. Later she, too, accepts her relationship with the Universe and begins to reframe her thinking accordingly.[2] Accepting Love makes us whole and unites us ultimately with the all-pervasive Force of the Divine.

## The Spiritual Energy of Love Lives Just Beneath the Surface of Our Lives

The search for our spiritual energy and the lessons it draws forth is no easier or more difficult than our search to tap an all-knowing level of our physical or emotional health. Our bodies, emotions, and spirits all have deeper levels that are beneath the most obvious personality or physical-symptoms levels. We must search to find what lives at these different depths.

Emotionally, we know the way we feel every day and the usual responses we make to those around us. We also know that a deeper, more loving level of feelings is sometimes available to us. We may also recognize that deep, painful feelings are also inside us, and even though we may want to forget these, they remain. Our bodies may seem fine, other than experiencing an occasional pain in one place or another; yet inside, out of our everyday awareness, we may be growing a tumor, or our blood vessels may be becoming so clogged we are about to have a heart attack—but we don't know it. It seems clear that to have better health and to understand what motivates and drives us, we need to discover the many aspects of the energy of Love that allow us an expanded perspective to explore the six major influences spiritual energy exerts in our lives. These influences are: Reflection, Partnership, Integration, Alignment, Rejuvenation, and Nourishment.

In order to understand our spiritual energy in these six major aspects we need to develop skills of intuition and deeper awareness through meditation or quiet periods of reflection that can educate us adequately to our own level of truth and to the influences of Love. As we seek greater understanding from the God-force, we can find the "energy snags" that hang us up spiritually. By learning to follow these energy snags into our physical bodies' symptoms and emotional bodies' feelings of loss, we find the imbalances of Love that produce disease and distress.

## Six Truths for All Living Things

We ask ourselves continually if we've found the truth, if we are doing enough to cure our diseases or heal our lives. Spiritual energy is elusive, and we are always asking ourselves if what we perceive in meditation is actually true or only our emotions talking to us. We experience the energy of Love in our lives in many different ways, and each has something important to tell us about ourselves and our inner health. I think of spiritual energy, Love, as similar to the air we breathe. When we are breathing normally we aren't concerned with the quality or content of the air. If we find ourselves in a room with insufficient oxygen, however, we very quickly feel panicked, and the quality of the air becomes of paramount importance because we fear for our very lives.

Our spiritual search should be no less dramatic. When we have people in our lives to love us, we don't question either the Universe's Love for us or our need for this energy of Love. But when life shifts beneath our feet and we lose Love from those around us, our health falters, our feelings fail to reassure us, our belief in God sags, and we fail to understand what we have done wrong.

No one is without Love by choice. Most people live on an emotional merry-go-round, forever searching for real Love and never finding it. Eventually, we give up and settle for Love in whatever ways we can get it. The search for Love as a universal energy requires us to think about Love in a different way—Love as the opportunity to grow into our own greatest potential while maintaining the balance of the whole. This definition of Love implies that we are responsible to ourselves to grow spiritually. At the same time we are responsible to support the growth of other living things in order to perpetuate the whole system. The energy of Love involves more than absorbing energy; it also requires our giving back so that ultimately the health of the entire system feeds back through us and all other living things to give Love and life.

The energy of Love is both a universal truth and a personal emotion. Because Love is universal, its influence touches all living things no matter where they live or what they look like. Love is a universal truth because it tells us and shows us through our life choices that when we act in support of the largest living system, we also support our own living systems. When we live in support of the spiritual energy of Love we also support and heal our bodies and emotional diseases and fears. Gerald Jampolsky, author of *Teach Only Love*, describes Love as "the total absence of fear and the basis for all attitudinal healing."[3]

As we approach the next millennium, we are being called to live with greater awareness of our own spiritual natures as well as our interrelationships with the God-source and all other living things. It is, therefore, essential that we consider the spiritual influences that all living things are touched by and that we as people are being called to acknowledge. In my work I have explored six influences of Love that form the spiritual energy blueprint for all life. And for each influence we'll look at the emotional responses that signal energy leaks in our lives and lead to impairment or disease in specific major systems or parts of our physical bodies. We'll also contrast a balanced emotional response with responses that drain our energy.

The six spiritual energy influences of Love (see Figure 1) give us the inner impulse that calls us to live in those ways that are most supportive of our individual spiritual growth and a balanced relationship with all other life. Any level of lasting healing requires our conscious use of these spiritual energy influences in order to live a balanced, healthy life in harmony with the God-source. When we can identify those influences we know we are out of balance with, we can assume that the corresponding physical systems and body parts nourished by those energy influences are at risk. If we already have a specific disease, or physical or emotional quandary or disturbance that we're aware of, then we can also trace it to the corresponding spiritual

### *Figure 1:*
## The Six Spiritual Energy Influences of Love

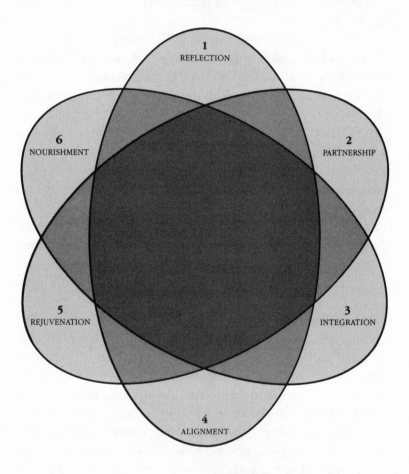

influence that affects its balance. Later on in the book we'll be discussing essential lifestyle shifts and choices we can make to correct the imbalances we've identified in our personal lives.

Earlier, I said we are being called to live with greater awareness of our interrelationships with "all living things." Perhaps this phrase needs clarification. I've defined "all living things" as those tangible individual elements of life, or larger systems of life composed of these elements, that are other than man-made. A rock, a flower, an animal, a worm, a bird, a microbe, and a molecule of water are all "living things." When we create products that are derivatives of living elements, such as a brick, a board, or clothing, then we are moving into a different relationship to energy. For purposes of this book, I'm suggesting that those elements that remain in their whole and original state, unaltered by humankind, are responsive to the spiritual energy influences of Love.

## Spiritual Energy Influence #1: Reflection

*All living things awaken eventually to the realization that they are aspects of Divine Love and thus live beyond any physical form.*

The energy of Reflection awakens us to our God-awareness, to the realization that the energy of Love is given from the God-source and again re-absorbed into its energy. All living things also recognize initially that their existence in any physical form is temporary and that it can and will change and become readjusted throughout eternity.

Obviously, not all forms of life meditate, but they do possess consciousness, meaning awareness of both their alignment with the God-source in the larger system of life and with their own individual identity. Every living thing senses that its time, in any form other than the pure state of spirit, is limited. Also accepted is that once the specific physical form dies, all energy is reunited with the larger God-system.

This is the truth that we know deep inside us but may have forgotten. Some level of ourselves knows that when we die we return to pure energy and that we continue to learn in a multitude of other ways, perhaps through additional incarnations into other physical forms. An individual cell within a muscle of a mouse has the same awareness of life and death as does a particle within a gaseous cloud in one of the rings around the planet Saturn—as does every human being.

## Balanced Emotional Response

When we have the Reflection aspect of spiritual energy in balance, we feel free to risk showing people the person we truly are by responding to life from our own self-worth and self-love. We are unafraid to try new and different things because we accept that we will have ample chances in this lifetime and others to respond to our challenges in a wide variety of ways.

## Emotional Responses that Signal Energy Leaks

- "If I say what I think, other people won't like me or will think I'm strange or different."
- "When my friends or spouse want me to go with them to do things that I really don't want to do, I never know how to tell them I don't want to go so that they won't get angry or feel hurt. I find myself just going along and feeling upset or just resigned to the fact that other people never do what I want."
- "I slant what I tell people, or tell them only half the truth, because I'm afraid they won't agree with me or support my needs."
- "My friend/colleague is so smug about her (or his)

accomplishments and always telling others how ter-
rific she (or he) is. What really makes me mad is
that people believe her (or him). Why can't they see
through that false facade?"

- "My feeling is you need to tell people exactly what
the situation is and be sure to hold them accountable
or they will always take the easy way out."

*Major Systems and Parts of Our Physical Bodies that Are
Influenced by the Energy of Reflection*

LYMPHATIC SYSTEM—supports our immune response to
disease and helps protect the body from invasion and
breakdown; also distributes the body's fluids.

*Body parts*—spleen, the lymphatic vessels, and the lymph.

## Spiritual Energy Influence #2: Partnership

*All living things bond initially and continually with the God-force.
The spiritual energy blueprint for all living things is to eventually
accept that Love is the primary component of bonding. This suggests that all living things seek bonds to encourage spiritual development in addition to procreation or furthering of their kind.*

All living things need relationships with others of their own
kind. We human beings know that to be happy we need many
kinds of relationships, and the spiritual energy of partnership
balances these essential needs. Today's physicists tell us we are
not the only living things that form bonds; intentional relationships exist both at the subatomic particle level and at the
whole-systems level, as evidenced by the development of certain patterns like those that produce the Earth's natural

resources of land, water, and an atmosphere allowing for human life. The patterns of life at every level form in support of directives from the God-source.

The implications for changes in human relationships suggest that we are being guided to participate in relationships with each other and with other elements of life differently, more lovingly, and in response to spiritual directives. While we have tended to spend time defining our spiritual connection with those we are intimate with, we now need also to define our spiritual bonds in all relationships and live in harmony with the Earth and all its myriad life forms. This spiritual energy of Partnership is drawing us toward accepting and giving Love as the basis for growing and healing personally and for helping to balance the entire God-system.

## Balanced Emotional Response

When we have the Partnership aspect of spiritual energy in balance, we are able to seek relationships based on our "awakened spirits" and our capacity to give and receive Love. We know that Love is the primary instrument of personal growth and that our lives will find meaning in relationships as we feel strengthened in our ability to honor our own spirits' initiatives. This means we are able to accept our spiritual guidance and allow its wisdom to direct our relationships.

## Emotional Responses that Signal Energy Leaks

- "It's difficult to develop serious relationships in which spirituality is also important to the other person; most of the men and women I meet are interested only in a good time."
- "My partner isn't interested in spirituality but doesn't mind if I am."
- "My partner doesn't understand my needs; he (or

she) takes for granted that I'll always be the way he
(or she) has known me in the past. My future in this
relationship looks pretty bleak."

- "I want a relationship with someone who always
understands my needs, is available to help me, and
appreciates all my struggles."

*Major Systems and Parts of Our Physical Bodies that Are*
*Influenced by the Energy of Partnership*
REPRODUCTIVE SYSTEM—functions to create new life and
to support the male and female organs that are essential for this purpose and for the purpose of deepening
the enjoyment in sexual intimacy.

*Body parts—in the male*: testes, seminal vesicles, penis,
urethra, prostate, and bulbourethral
glands.
*in the female*: the ovaries, Fallopian
tubes, uterus, vagina, and vulva plus
breasts.

CIRCULATORY SYSTEM—distributes essential life-supporting
ingredients to the body and collects others for
elimination.
*Body parts*—heart, blood vessels, and blood.

## Spiritual Energy Influence #3: Integration

*All living things have an inner integrity that is composed of*
*spirit within a physical form. Each living system will come to*
*know and honor its unique presence and function through experi-*
*ences within specific living environments.*

In watching a dancer or athlete, we imagine the millions of actions and responses, both mental and physical,

required to achieve the desired result of running a race or performing a pirouette in ballet. This total mental and physical absorption and single-minded focus produces "peak performances." Love gives all living things the opportunity for continuous peak experiences when they honor the harmony of their bodies and harmony of their minds with their spirits. The deeper self, the spirit, initiates a "spiritual beat" that the other parts of the body and mind must match and support. When the body and mind forget or block out this spiritual beat, inner harmony breaks down.

Integration is an internal influence that allows our systems to work effectively with their individual parts to create health and harmony. When our mental or feeling aspects are in alignment with this aspect of spiritual energy, our physical bodies work optimally. The energy of Integration creates an inner harmony that is essential to the balanced functioning of our individual lives.

*Balanced Emotional Response*
When we have the Integration aspect of spiritual energy in balance, we are able to appreciate the spiritual, emotional, and physical qualities of our being and to improve communication between our spirits and our feelings, our feelings and our bodies, and our spirits and our bodies. We are able to do these things to further an inner harmony that we realize is essential for our health and our appreciation of life.

*Emotional Responses that Signal Energy Leaks*
- "I usually feel overwhelmed with life, as if I have so much to do and not enough time in which to do it. I often feel a knot in my stomach, and I know I'm pushing myself too hard."
- "I feel out of touch with any personal relationship

with the God-source. I'm not sure what I even believe about God.

- "I never have the time to sit down and read the books I've bought to try and make some sense out of my life."
- "I feel disconnected from my body."
- "I don't like my body—it's let me down."
- "I feel as if I could fly apart into a million pieces."

*Major Systems and Parts of Our Physical Bodies that Are Influenced by the Energy of Integration*

SENSORY PARTS—composed of receptors that provide awareness of an individual's living environment.

*Body parts*—eyes, ears, and nose (mouth and tongue, while also sensory parts of the body, are listed under #6, Nourishment).

SKELETAL SYSTEM—supports, protects, and encourages movement of the physical frame.

*Body parts*—bones, and the connective tissues that tie them together.

MUSCULAR SYSTEM—causes movement and helps to maintain and support the physical frame.

*Body parts*—muscles, such as in the biceps, and those like the muscular lining of the stomach.

TISSUES—the cells and groups of cells arranged to form tissues that support and protect the body.

*Body parts*—epithelial or boundary tissues, such as the skin, the digestive tube; connective tissue that connects, insulates, and forms protective sheaths that are continuous throughout the body; muscular tissue that

allows for parts of the body to contract,
thus allowing for breathing, beating of the
heart, movement of parts of the alimentary canal, as well as other viscera including
blood and lymph vessels; nerve tissue that
is able to respond to stimulation and to
transmit the stimuli or nerve impulses to
other cells;  membranes that are thin
expansions of tissues serving as linings
and coverings of the body.

## Spiritual Energy Influence #4:  Alignment

*All living things are encouraged to realize that the changes
in their lives reflect essential changes of universal energy from
the God-source, and that this energy is meant to help them
clarify their own purpose for living.*

Every living thing has a purpose, and all living things
except human beings are at some level fully aware of their
charge here on the Earth.  All aspects of a banana tree, for
instance, come together in support and harmony to create a
specific kind of fruit, a certain kind of leafy vegetation,
bark, and roots—all of which together support the produc-
tion of fruit that furthers the growth and development of a
tree.  Likewise, each living element grows as an essential
part of the entire God-force.  Nothing extraneous exists
within the system; all is essential, just as all the parts of our
physical and emotional bodies are essential to help the
whole body operate well.

All living things adjust to immediate environmental
changes, such as heat or cold, but ultimately, the purpose
of each level of life responds more directly to the largest

level of life—the God-force—and the energy of Love. While all living things are aware that they function in relationship to this greater force, mass evolutionary shifts and jumps happen in accordance with spiritual factors rather than exclusively environmental ones. As the needs of the Divine system change to accommodate its myriad ancillary systems, so survival of any person, species, culture, or planet depends on its ability to absorb and maintain an appropriate level of Love.

### Balanced Emotional Response

When we have the Alignment aspect of spiritual energy in balance, we are able to accommodate the changes in our lives because we know they bring us ever closer to our purposes for living. We accept that we are unique in all of the universe and that we have a right to fulfilling lives. We accept that we seek happiness through the search and clarification of our purpose, knowing that it stems from Divine Love.

### Emotional Responses that Signal Energy Leaks

- "I'm not sure what I'm really supposed to be doing with my life."
- "Other people seem to know the ways to get what they want—I never know if I should move or change jobs, or what the problem is."
- "Change frightens me, and I don't adjust well to things being different. It's hard for me to give away old clothes or furniture. I like routines, and it's upsetting when people want to do things that aren't part of the norm."

*Major Systems and Parts of Our Physical Bodies that Are Influenced by the Energy of Alignment.*

NERVOUS SYSTEM—coordinates various nerve impulses to allow an individual to understand and relate appropriately to his or her environment.

*Body parts*—brain, spinal cord, ganglia, nerve fibers, and sensory and motor terminals.

ENDOCRINE SYSTEM—maintains equilibrium through the distribution of specific secretions that affect functioning of cells, organs, and tissues.

*Body parts*—thyroid, parathyroid, pituitary, adrenals, portions of glands with ducts like Islands of Langerhans in the pancreas, portions of the ovaries and testes, and the pineal gland.

## Spiritual Energy Truth #5: Rejuvenation

*All living things participate in cycles within physical life that imitate the larger cycles of life and death. These cycles are spiritually-ordered, encouraging the alternation between periods of contraction or focused attention and those of rest and relaxation.*

The specific energy put into each cycle of life changes to create balance. All living things have seasons or periods in which attention or contraction is balanced by relaxation and Rejuvenation. Just as animals gather food some of the time, play some of the time, eat, sleep, and procreate some of the time, humans should also vary their activities according to the cycles of living, which are essential to the quality of joy in human life and to our longevity.

We humans are the only living things that inadvertently maintain continual levels of attention; we call this stress. Our inability to play, laugh, enjoy life in its natural beauty shortens our lives and cuts down on our enjoyment. Whether or not we understand life cycles at the sub-atomic level, we can accept that the states of focused attention are no more important than those of relaxation. Theoretically, if we could absorb enough Love by balancing our times of attention and relaxation, our physical body would never die.

## *Balanced Emotional Response*

When we have the Rejuvenation aspect of spiritual energy in balance, we are able to accept the cycles of our lives knowing that they have a basis in Love. Rejuvenation enables us to accept the times of struggle as well as those of joy; we are able to work and attend to our business as well as we can and then relax, trusting that our intentions that are grounded in Love are continuing to direct our efforts.

## *Emotional Responses that Signal Energy Leaks*

- "It's very hard for me to relax. When I sit down I always feel that there are other things I must do."
- "I've forgotten how to play. I've been serious for so long and 'responsible' from such an early age that I feel awkward when I'm given opportunities to do things just for myself."
- "I worry a lot. Sometimes I wake up early, and by the time I'm showered and ready for breakfast I'm already tired from all the worrying."
- "I'm afraid that if I let down and relax at work that my boss will promote someone else. He (or she) thinks that when we are thinking about work all the time and are doing extra work at home that these are the signs of a truly committed person."

*Major Systems and Parts of Our Physical Bodies that Are Influenced by the Energy of Rejuvenation*

RESPIRATORY SYSTEM—provides oxygen and gets rid of carbon dioxide.

*Body parts*—nose, pharynx, larynx, trachea, bronchi, and lungs.

EXCRETORY SYSTEM—eliminates waste from cell activity.

*Body parts*—urinary organs such as the kidneys, ureters, bladder, urethra, and the skin.

## Spiritual Energy Influence #6: Nourishment

*All living things eventually accept that they are nourished most significantly by Love. While aspects of living need many kinds of nourishment, only nourishment that is aligned with the spiritual intention of perpetuating Love is able to fully heal or nourish.*

We know the ways living things need physical food and water, and some also need air to live on the Earth. Yet the energy of Love provides a balance to the tissues and fibers of our lives in ways that are so little understood that we all but overlook this ingredient as a factor in healing.

Just as we humans are nourished by relationships and loving acceptance and encouragement from others, so are all other living things. A tree knows the difference between attack and appreciation; an animal thrives on loving attention and dies with neglect. Who knows? We may eventually come to the place where we can live on Love alone.

*Balanced Emotional Response*

When we have the Nourishment aspect of spiritual energy

in balance, we are able to find fulfillment in our lives. We are comfortable making the choices that feel satisfying to our bodies, our emotions, our intellects, and our spirits. We are able to make our own choices regarding our lifestyle needs and to seek inner awareness when questioning the value of those things that we seek nourishment from.

*Emotional Responses that Signal Energy Leaks*
- "I seem to have no will power when it comes to food."
- "I have trouble staying with a new routine even though I know it will make me healthier."
- "I'm always worried about having enough money. I tell myself that money isn't really the issue, but I can't stop thinking that if I had more money I'd be so much happier."

*Major Systems and Parts of Our Physical Bodies that Are Influenced by the Energy of Nourishment*
DIGESTIVE SYSTEM—receives and digests food by absorbing into the body what it needs to support metabolism and the physical and emotional bodily functions.

*Body parts*—alimentary canal, including the mouth, tongue, salivary glands and teeth, pharynx, esophagus, stomach, small and large intestine, pancreas, and liver.

## The Energy of Your Spirit

Healing occurs when our spiritual energy is balanced within us and when this energy is balanced in our bodies, our emotions, and our lifestyles. The spiritual energy of Love is ever-present with us, but we must choose to allow it into our lives, and we must make the on-going choices for our lives that keep it present. Like a hungry fish swimming in a pond filled with algae and worms, if we don't open our mouths, we will, symbolically, starve to death.

Thus does the energy of Love flow into our bodies through these six influences of spirit: Reflection, Partnership, Integration, Alignment, Rejuvenation, and Nourishment. All these influences serve to nourish and support our relationship with other living things and with the God-force. Love as energy flows where it is drawn to us by our intention to be of service in those ways that affirm life's wholeness. Becoming aware of other living things and being compassionate in our actions are both essential in order to draw spiritual energy into our lives. Every way that we respond to life in affirming the ingredients of wholeness and in preserving diversity, we authenticate Love and draw it into our lives. Each way we think, feel, and act that denigrates or destroys cuts us off from life and diminishes our supply of Love. As we appreciate the types of balance offered us by each spiritual influence, we can better grasp our present physical and emotional "power outages" that result in disease or distress.

## Rediscovering the Authentic Power of Love

When we are in crisis we need to feel the reassurance of Divine Love. We want to feel loved and protected beyond the reaches of disease, loss, divorce, death, or any sort of fear. We expect that when God helps or blesses us the misery will disappear. But unknowingly, we often hold on to the struggle. To become whole we must separate those beliefs and identities that belong only to physical life from those that are of spirit. When we make these essential distinctions we allow our bodies and our emotions to find and believe in the unifying force of our spirits. The one consistent truth is that Divine Love is drawn specifically into our lives to expand our capacity to love.

I imagine a soul to resemble a finely-tooled silver chalice. When we are born we have the capability of filling our chalices with Love. The God-force initially supplies us with just enough Love to get us safely into this life; from then on, we are each responsible for gathering the energy of Love ourselves. The God-force doesn't guarantee that we will fill our silver soul-chalices, only that we will have opportunities every day to try.

The most crucial experience any of us can have—must have—is to be loved. Without exception, we can grow in health and compassion only in discovering the God-force at work in our lives. Healing occurs in the name of Love. And all our journeys, whether or not we accept it consciously, are to rediscover the authentic power and meaning of the energy of Love.

## Your Universal Purpose for Being

We come into this life alone, and we leave it alone. I believe we are each on the Earth on assignment, to find and use Love and to discover the power of our spirits to harmonize our bodies and minds in ways that comfort us and make us whole. This is a time to change and to grow, and to do this we need to live each moment in an awareness of Love. Each moment of life can be a blessing, not because of what we have accomplished or the material possessions we've acquired but because we are in harmonious relationship with the Divine and all other living things.

Love generated intentionally with the God-force grows

more quickly than any other emotion. It is the grandmother of all emotions. This Love heals, helps us in even unseen ways, and can be given away without being lost. When this Love meets disease, the disease lessens. When this Love meets pain, the pain leaves. Love is the answer to whatever the problem is. As we release our doubts, our lack of belief, our fear and pain, we are rejuvenated. When we appreciate our courage and tenacity, our strength and will, we can also believe in our capacity to change and heal. These powerful and affirming feelings about ourselves are reflections of Divine Love.

Often, we feel that others are not as sensitive to our struggle as they should be. Or perhaps they seem unable to give us the kind of loving attention that we feel we need. We can be nurtured by other people's Love even when it is incomplete, needy, smothering, or demanding. When we love ourselves we can absorb the best of Love from other people and leave the rest.

## Love: The Essential Element for Healing

We are all capable of healing and of dismantling the barricades erected among the body, mind, and spirit even though we may have stopped giving ourselves the Love we need. At such a time we can begin to heal. Without Love we are unable to hold onto the energy we are building; our energy reserves are dissipated easily and dramatically and take time to rebuild.

The world of spiritual energy is the world of the God-force and its Love. The physical world responds to matter, but it is the spiritual world that initiates what matter will become.

Our silver soul-chalices can hold Love and healing energy whenever we decide that we are ready to make the effort to honor the requests for Love coming from ourselves and from all other living aspects of the God-force. As we become reacquainted with our spiritual selves, we recognize more readily the call to love someone or something else when it comes to us. Finally, we can feel Love in more symbolic and diverse ways when we need to respond to groups of people or entire ecosystems that are calling for the same Love. Humanity's greatest hope for the future lies in our potential, individually, to learn to love so that we use this expansive energy to heal all levels of life. We are each part of this extravaganza of life on the planet and its widely divergent life forms. We find meaning in one way or another from the simple act of loving.

## NOTES

1. Joan Borysenko, *Guilt is the Teacher, Love is the Lesson* (New York, NY: Warner Books, 1990), p. 128.

2. Shirley MacLaine, *Out on a Limb* (New York, NY: Bantam, 1983).

3. Gerald G. Jampolsky, *Teach Only Love* (New York, NY: Bantam Books, 1983), p. xii.

# 4 Preparing Yourself to Heal

*To surrender means to acquiesce and allow,*
*to cease resistance and acknowledge that*
*perhaps the purpose of your life isn't in what*
*you've accomplished but in what intention you've*
*brought to the task.*

When our lives are in disarray and distress, we want to do the things that can make it right and get us back on our feet. We know that the responsibility is ours, and through the long nights and early morning hours we spend many a moment assessing the positive and negative aspects of our situations and our chances to heal our lives or sustain them in the ways we want. Those early morning hours are extremely poignant times. Maybe it's the darkness that is disorienting—we can't see our bodies—and we imagine what it would be like to be a spirit without a body. If we ever considered suicide, this is the time we think about it.

We are alone while our loved ones sleep on peacefully. We keep the early morning vigil by ourselves. More people die in the early morning hours than at any other time of the day or night. I imagine that in these early hours more people also surrender to a higher wisdom and thus find the grit that ultimately becomes their pearl.

In order to heal we know that serious mental, spiritual, and physical work must be undertaken. We may feel like a runner beginning a marathon and wondering if we'll be able to finish. No one knows, and perhaps whether we complete the race isn't even significant. The runner will never accomplish the distance unless she is able to pay close attention to the job of putting one foot down in front of the other.

Each of us is running his or her own race, alone and yet not alone. No one else can understand what we feel. Others see only what we show them: they see the moods and the countenance we want them to see. They don't know what we feel. They are a million miles away from our fear. Always in the back of our minds lingers the reality of our situation. Through the dinner conversation, across the expanse of daily chores—it's always waiting there to tell us we may not make it, or we may be unable to do what is required to get better.

In some ways preparing to heal is like learning to write. About the time we're feeling as if we've really accomplished something, our inner voice, our "editor," pipes up to erode our confidence. In *Wild Mind,*[1] author Natalie Goldberg talks about this "inner editor" and the ways to circumvent this destructive and distracting dialogue that immobilizes and undermines our efforts and our confidence. Yet we can sometimes find the courage to start on the path up the mountain we must climb, the mountain that is in our path. One way to circumvent this destructive inner voice and step out on the path is to find another truth that lies behind the voice. We can learn to write, talk, and meditate through this voice of our inner editor so that she has less influence on us.

We transcend this voice of our past and our limitations by building assurance in a newly-emerging intuitive self, who believes in rules that have a greater reach and capacity to heal than those accepted by our editor voice. We assume other people were never disturbed by an inner voice the way we are and that they never felt the fear we do. We assume others have confronted their own mountains and never once faltered or looked back. That isn't true. Acting from inner courage doesn't mean you aren't afraid, only that you overcome the fear—you tap something else within you that allows you to overcome the fear, or at least neutralize it. This is the healing journey to wholeness that you have undertaken. You aren't expected to be unafraid; the challenge is to raise your gaze above the fear and to embrace the quality of your life and your contribution to life each moment of each day.

## Assessing Your Life and Weighing Your Choices

You may feel that, no matter the size of this mountain in your path, it is time to get set up to heal. To do this requires assessing the day-to-day practices, relationships, habits, and attitudes that hold you to a way of living that you want to break free of. This initial level of preparation is important and also easily understood. Healing requires using your good sense, your intuition, your belief in yourself and in those you invite into your life. Begin as you can, where you can, and accept the level of change that each new wave of effort brings. As in the children's story of *The Little Engine That Could*, you'll build your own level of steam slowly but surely.

The days ahead in your journey toward wholeness and spiritual discovery will awaken a part of you that may never have been in charge before. One day you'll feel as if you have everything under control, and then a trip to the oncologist, the therapist, or your former spouse will shatter your resolve, and you'll be tossed into the doldrums, feeling you've made no progress whatsoever.

Personal growth is measured in the reframing of your life picture. Each time you have a setback, the pieces of your life are broken apart, and you are required to heal in a different way. Although this is frightening and unpleasant, it is essential. We thrive on the familiar, but now you are scrutinizing everything in your life with a different eye. A major step in your healing requires recognizing the aspects of your personal behavior and attitudes that are beneficial and those that are deleterious. You have all the time you need to make the change in attitude that requires you to address the circumstances of your life in some way. You can take that time to consider all your options, to weigh all your choices. Often, merely accepting that you have the power to make different choices shifts the healing balance in your favor.

## Taking Charge of Your Own Healing

What happens when what you think you should do conflicts with what your spouse, family, or children want you to do? At such times we're not sure whose wishes we should follow. Sometimes we let others make our decisions because doing so keeps the peace. Sometimes we just want others to make the decisions for us because we're ambiguous about our own needs. Sometimes we are afraid of our own power and hesitate to let it out of the box. We may sense that, if we take over our own healing programs, our most immediately supporting relationships will be threatened.

I know a woman who has inoperable cancer. She is eighty years old and feels she's led a good life. Her husband can't let her die. He sits in on every conversation that she has. He's desperate to be needed and in control of her life. He is an atheist, and so he intercedes in, and dismisses, any conversations she has with others that might open doors to questioning her beliefs. She doesn't want to upset him and in her present weakened state is grateful for his care and feels she is in no position to do other than she's doing. Essentially, she's closed off her own choices.

In caring for yourself it is essential that you recognize that you have choices in everything you do, think, and feel. If you choose to follow a specific course of action, it becomes an asset in your column of positive healing initiatives. When you fume privately and push away the feelings that you are afraid to acknowledge, then you keep disease and disability alive in your life.

If you find that you must go to the hospital for surgery, to a convalescent home to recuperate, to one of your children's homes to live, or to a nursing home, you can do so with your inner power and confidence intact if you fit the choice that you are about to make with the wisdom of your best thinking. Also involved is the reality of your situation.

A client of mine went to the hospital to have major abdominal surgery for cancer. When she'd had previous operations, she felt helpless and powerless in the hospital: she felt she had no "say" in what was done to her and that no one really cared or asked for her opinion. This time she and I talked at great length about the difference between being the victim in the situation and taking charge. She decided that, rather than drop everything to rush to "Admittance" the first time someone called to say a bed was vacant, she would arrange the date of the surgery at a time that was convenient for her, and she felt right about doing that. She asked the surgeon specific questions about the surgery, the prognosis, the medication, and the recuperation period. Most significant, she decided whether or not she wanted the surgery in the first place. She decided she did, and so she was taking this initiative because she felt it would give her the time necessary to work on the spiritual levels of healing that required her full attention.

When she went to the hospital she took with her a small tote bag of items that made her feel in control of her life. She took mementos of her family, a pillow that was soft and satiny and felt soothing next to her face, a funny cartoon, a book of meditations, and subliminal and talking tapes on healing. She felt peaceful when she went into the hospital. She had taken charge of her life to the degree that she could, and the result was a positive experience in the hospital and a speedier than normal recovery. Instead of feeling as if she'd been disempowered by the experience, she felt that she had participated in it on her terms.

Healing does not always require such radical approaches as surgery, of course. People come forward daily sharing the procedures, medicines, remedies, and healing methods that have reduced pain, even eliminated tumors, and helped others regain their health, often in miraculous ways. This should show us that we can just about heal with grape leaves if the power of our spirits fully endorses the procedure. While certain medical interventions are more difficult to recover from, and some leave us more debilitated than

others, we do have a wide variety of choices. We can successfully "mix and match" our approaches so that they
include ways to address our emotional needs, our spiritual
relationship with a God-force or larger living system, and
the physical requirements we believe can most help us heal.

The recurrence rate of disease and the long haul of chronic
trauma, emotional or physical, puts severe stress on our lives
and our relationships. When diseases recur after we think
we've finished with them, it is hard to accept that healing is a
process and that this form of challenge may be the form our
spiritual work will take over the years. If we have serious
relationship or family problems that never seem to heal but
remain painful and open wounds emotionally, then accepting
these avenues as our teachers allows us each day to focus less
on getting somewhere and more on the quality of our
thoughts, responses, and questions. Healing is truly a process
we take on at birth. As we grow through life we are on the
one hand feeling defined by our life experiences and on the
other seeking to transcend these limits by ascribing to a spiritual philosophy of unlimited potential.

## To Leave or Not to Leave a Relationship

Most people who eventually leave a marriage or were themselves left saw the change coming but were helpless to alter
the outcome. We can both love and hate at the same time:
love a person with whom we've spent many years but hate
his or her attitudes, actions, or responses to our needs.
Relationships teach us so much about ourselves. If we do
get a divorce, we're often shocked to discover that even
though the person we leave may be gone the issues that we
abhorred are still very present.

We are meant to learn from our partners. This means

accepting that we are different human beings with diverse, possibly complementary personalities and beliefs, and both of us have our own inner work to do. Men often expect women to be the intuitive and nurturing ones, and women often expect men to be the primary breadwinners. This false expectancy is obviously changing as both adults work, both raise children, and both learn the art and necessity of nurturing with solid emotional support and communication skills.

There is no easy answer to the dilemma of whether or not to leave a marriage or long-standing relationship. Ultimately, I've found that the force of our inner feelings pushes us toward crescendos and solutions even against our wishes. Our relationships are either gaining momentum or losing it; the energy of partnership doesn't remain static for any of us. We may think we can go on with life and our unhappy relationships by just ignoring the red flags of trouble. But ultimately we either get sick, fall in love with someone else, or break the stalemate in some other way.

If you decide to leave a relationship, try to do as much of the personal work as possible, both alone and jointly. Try to be open with your feelings and resist blaming each other. I've found that if we stick to talking about our perceptions in terms of "me" or "I," then the other person is able to hear, accept, and perhaps learn from what we are saying. If we say "you," then we are into the blame game, and the anger and frustration of the discussion satisfies no one. We humans are all learning that the art of communication requires us to present what we feel is true, listen attentively and openly to what others are saying is true for them, and make determinations based on our "best selves" rather than our "needy selves."

We often stay in an obviously or subtly abusive relationship because we've gotten used to it, we don't know anything else, we aren't sure we can support ourselves and our children on our own, we're afraid to leave for fear of real or implied retaliation, or we just don't know how to get out of it. If we are in an emotionally or physically abusive relationship, then the sooner we can call it by this name the more easily we will be able to remove ourselves and perhaps our children to safer ground or take other measures to get professional help. Women often allow others to abuse them by feeling that they deserve to be abused, or that they don't realize relationships can be different. If you even wonder whether your partner's responses are out of line, then they probably are.

If your partner is insensitive to your needs, insisting that your needs or demands are wrong, stop and ask yourself if this feels true. A woman trying to heal from cancer announced to me recently that her boyfriend used to go to the other end of the living room to smoke and insisted that putting this much distance between them was good enough. She was able to temporarily break off the relationship to give herself a little time to question his behavior and her needs for healing.

## Put Your "Inner Sensing" to Work

Everyone has an ability to sense some aspect of truth beyond the normal five-senses reality, and we apply this sensing to different fields of interest. Some might use their sense to predict when it will snow, or where the fish are biting, or how to carve away the parts of a block of granite that aren't to be part of a sculpture. Our healing is increased through our ability to sense our inner health or specific inner imbalances. When we are seriously ill or upset, we spend a great deal of time worrying rather than learning to sense our needs, fears, and healing potential.  When we seek specific information inside of us through meditation or prayer, we then have specific information or thoughts that we can put to work for our healing.  Worry can cease, and productive action can begin.

Another word for sensing that we are more familiar with is *intuiting*.  Listening to our inner voice through our intuition helps us direct our energy in the most productive ways.  The voice of our intuition, inner sensing, is different from our fears that tell us to pretend that our situation will vanish without attention or effective treatment, or that a serious problem may not really be present.

In healing we are trying to apply our intuitive perceptions to our bodies and emotions to speed their recovery and regain health.  Often, we feel that while we have intuitive skill in other aspects of our lives, we are unable to "listen" to what our organs or circumstances in our lives are really telling us.  A man who was a portrait painter was convinced that he had no intuitive skill when it came to assessing his state of health or disease.  Yet when he talked about his painting he noted that he could paint the muscles, the nerves, and marvelously subtle expressions because he simply "felt" what these parts of a person's face were saying to him.  This intuition of the portrait painter is exactly the same inner sense we work with ultimately in asking our bodies, our emotions, and our spirits to help us understand their needs and the ways we can help their search for balance.

## Finding the Most Appropriate Healing Approaches

A common complaint from people who are trying to make choices for healing care is that there are simply too many healing approaches to choose from.  The abundance of holistic and traditional medical approaches to the healing of disease and to the support of one's emotional or spiritual needs can be bewildering.

We are able to consider only a few methods of treatment at one time. Author Linda Frazer Fleming, in *Releasing Arthritis: The Seven Year Plan*,[2] describes the way she made a list of fifteen types of healing approaches that she wanted to try in her effort to heal. She gave herself five years to cover all of them by taking one at a time and making an honest attempt to give each a try. Making a plan and trying those methods you are interested in can open you to teachers and practitioners who are able to facilitate your healing journey.

If you have a situation that demands immediate attention, then you would be well to pick only a few approaches for consideration and learn about each one separately. A client of mine went to three health-care practitioners in two days. She talked first to a person teaching a Macrobiotic approach to nutrition. Then she went to a man who worked with body electricity and balancing of the energy fields. Finally, she met with an Anthroposophic physician to discuss mistletoe injections. By this time she was so confused and depressed that she felt thoroughly overwhelmed. I've found that the most productive avenues a person can pursue come from those friends or family members whose opinions you trust. Your own initiatives are important, but choose only a few to work on at any one time. This approach will offer you enough of a sampling of what you really need to explore.


## Dealing with Your Health Caregivers, Including Physicians

Talking honestly with your own medical practitioners presents you with a different set of challenges. Many people are intimidated by most physicians and are afraid that they will be put off by questioning either their choice of treatment for us or our desire to add other methods to their prescribed treatment of choice. And well they may be. But it's important that you are your own best advocate; no one is going to care as much about you or your problems or the quality of your life as you are.

Most people like and admire their doctors and are afraid of getting on their wrong side. One woman felt that her doctor would reject her if she decided to try alternative treatments before agreeing to his suggested chemotherapy. We have to pick our own way through this potential minefield. But if we accept that we and they are trying to do what is best for us, then when we apply our own inner guidance and come to decisions we can trust we may feel more confident in initiating potentially gritty discussion. Many times people are worried that they should have done something other than what they've tried. My feeling is that the quality of the effort you put into whatever you do is the most important element.

## Getting Even versus Getting Better

We've been raised on the belief that if something goes wrong, someone is always to blame. If the dishwasher breaks repeatedly, we call the repairman back, refusing to pay the bill until it's fixed. If we sustain a neck injury in an automobile accident, our insurance company sues the other driver's insurance company. There is a thin line between assuming a pro-active attitude that promotes our healing and blaming others for our situation.

We need to think twice, for instance, about entering into

situations that embroil us in unending and counterproductive litigation at a time when we need our full attention on our healing. Sometimes we feel that we need to "get that person, or make him (or her) pay." The negative energy effect of this "get even" attitude can be lethal. If the name of the game in healing is accepting responsibility for our choices and the outcomes these produce, then handing our problem to someone else to solve won't help us get better.

The more aspects of our lives that we handle ourselves as opposed to farming them out to others, the better off we are. When we sidestep confronting someone about that person's handling of a situation important to us, we give away our power. We in effect become the victim, the one acted on rather than doing the acting or making the decisions. All too often, this predicament translates a year or two later into disease or breakdown.

A friend of mine lost her elderly aunt in an unfortunate way, but her handling of the situation gave her back her inner power. Just prior to her demise, the aunt had been recovering successfully from major surgery and had returned to her nursing home, only to have an attendant fail to pull up the guard rail on her bed. The aunt became disoriented, tried to stand up, fell, and broke her hip. The accident's complications led to a painful and protracted death.

My friend was horrified and certainly had grounds for a lawsuit, yet she chose, instead, to go to the nursing home and talk to both the administrator and the nurse who was in charge the day of the accident. My friend told them that although the case was one of obvious negligence, she also understood that mistakes did happen. In the ensuing conversation she told them that her aunt had, until the time of the accident, felt loved and taken care of by the staff, and that she was sure that, like her, they felt very badly about this needless tragedy. The look on the young nurse's face told my friend that this experience was already imprinted indelibly on this woman's life. My friend was also firm about expecting the nursing home to pay the costs of the hospitalization.

In this situation, anywhere along the way the dialogue could have broken down, and a lawsuit could have ensued. But the effort to work things out person-to-person and face-to-face allows us the satisfaction of telling people the way we feel and also hearing the way they feel. This is ultimately much more personally empowering and healing.

Lingering feelings of blame are corrosive to our bodies and our emotional well-being. Winning or losing has nothing to do with our reclaiming our emotional power; staying involved does. When we do sit down and talk with the individuals we blame for our loss, we may discover that they are not the ogres we assumed or wanted to believe. Of course, this discovery brings us around full circle to saying, "Well, if this person isn't a bad person, then who is it I'm blaming?" Often, we blame ourselves for not taking action in a way that could have—or we think might have— made a difference. Or we blame life and want someone to pay for our loss. Accepting that things do happen beyond our control is perhaps healthier for us in the long run than insisting that someone be punished.

The point of dealing directly with people is to upgrade the quality of our responses and thus improve the overall level of exchange. This method of interacting leaves both parties free of long-term emotional scars. When we choose to respond from our own inner power, we lift the level of the potential solution because we've used fairness, right action, compassion, and honor. When our actions arise only from our anger and our need to retaliate, we've missed the opportunity to reinforce those beliefs that will leave us a whole person after the situation is finally resolved.

Our biggest challenge in saying that we accept a different, more compassionate belief system is that we are then also expected to act within that belief system.

## Remaining Flexible in the Face of Change

Moving with the forces of change is essential to surviving in a meaningful way. When we are flexible we flow with the challenges of life. When we're rigid, we break emotionally and/or physically. The physical circumstances of our lives require us to learn spiritually while at the same time accepting that we are part of a larger God-ordered system of life. Being willing and able to accept changing perceptions of our situation helps us grow, learn, and heal. We are living within an unpredictable Earth-School environment, and we are also in a physical world with physical laws that apply. If we walk in front of a moving car we will be hit, and perhaps with very serious results. Yet learning can always be gleaned from the experiences that help us lift our gaze and our determination from the physical to the spiritual level of living. We gain flexibility as we change our perception of our situation and consider new ways in which we can heal it.

We spend a great deal of time alone when we are sick or upset. Even though we are working spiritually to understand our situations, we may feel deeply lonely even if we are sharing the house with others. When loss threatens our lives we are the ones acutely aware of our own immortality and vulnerability. No matter the intentions of others to help, it is our own spiritual beliefs that are being tested and cracked open. When we are in spiritual crisis we want the Universe to show itself to us in a real way. "If only God could hold me when I'm afraid and feeling deserted," said a woman beginning her healing journey, "then I'd be sure that there really is a God and He or She knows me." The God-force becomes a living force in our healing as we take time to explore what we feel is being required of us. We are aligned with the Love of the Universe, and from this we draw our strength. We will need to learn that a flexible approach to living allows us to accept all that we are unable to change at this present moment and to change those things that we are able to change.

## Events Happen for a Reason

When we are healthy we expect a positive momentum to carry us forward. Yet we find the God-force in a more intimate way when we are in serious straits. When the ordinary routines of our lives are scattered by change, we are challenged to find God in more than the rhetoric on the written page or the passive image in a picture. We are challenged to find the God of our inner being that can sustain us in this struggle.

"God hurts, too, when I hurt, and I know She or He wants me to get stronger," said a woman who had found the way she could best appreciate the God-force in her life. If you are sincerely searching for the Universe in your life and for the answers that brought you to this place of dramatic change, then assume that the circumstances, encounters, opportunities, materials, and people that come into your life are present on purpose to offer you the assurance that you are aligned with a larger system of life. When you're pushing for understanding, there are no accidents.

The power of our prayers and meditations attract to us situations that can help us learn and recover. As we translate the ways in which Divinity is actually, noticeably, clearly, and definitely a true and present force in our lives, we begin to believe that a new beginning is possible.

## A Future Worth Living for

We' don't know, of course, why some people live and others die, why some heal with a certain treatment and others don't, but observation does tell us that when a person heals, certain factors are always present. A major factor that I've observed is that a person is able to identify a desire for a future, and that this future is worth living for.

In order to heal, we need to be returning to a life that offers us something substantially different from and better than what we have presently or that we've had in the past. Our living environment and emotional atmosphere need to be compatible with the growth we are experiencing through conscious work with our disease or loss. We heal not from a rational understanding of things we might want to do or have, or even from an emotional attachment to the people we love; the reason we heal is that we want to accomplish something that deals with our deepest spiritual purpose for life. Something truly significant remains for us to do. The question becomes, "How do we find or refine this authentic purpose for which we've been born?"

At every workshop and spiritual gathering I hear people lament their lack of understanding about their life purposes. Our purpose in life isn't a package that falls from the sky when we utter the magic word; it has always been with us, and we've seen it in various guises throughout our lives as we've helped or been of service in some way. Our purpose is so close to us that the clues we see go unnoticed, or we take them for granted, assuming them to be something else. Our purpose is tied to the means through which we are of service to the larger system, helping to build and maintain harmony within this hologram. Our future will emerge as we take one step at a time, moving with assurance as far as we can and then awaiting the inner feeling of energy and presence that spurs us to take the next step. Our job is to believe that we can accomplish what we will be intuitively shown, and that the energy and skill and ability we will need to accomplish our work is being awakened within us.

## Engaging Your Will Power for Healing

Will power is a more powerful and expanded version of our egos. We need our egos to help us live at the personality level. Our egos help us identify and meet our physical and emotional needs. Our spirits, however, convert simple ego to a more complex energy that is will power. Will power is the force of our spirits that is essential in healing ourselves or helping others heal. Will power exerts a more pervasive force on the body and emotions, and it isn't afraid of being extinguished by change. If our will power is engaged, we can face the most dismal and fearful situations and change successfully. Will power can't be created artificially. We must search for it through our own spiritual experience of rediscovering the God-force. We must search for it more vigorously when we are in spiritual crisis.

While we are intent upon eliminating pain and trauma in our lives, we learn the most when our needs are not being met or we have been stymied in some significant way. I've discovered that healing doesn't mean taking away the trauma or pain, it means allowing individuals the opportunity to work through it themselves, with our support. When we learn a process that we can duplicate, we know that we can survive. Healing requires that we experiment with the energy available to us. We all know the flush of feeling the strength of our convictions, the strength that lets us know we can survive the changes we must make. When we have these rushes of tangible energy, we know that our spirits are awake and well and we are engaging our will power to heal.

## NOTES

1. Natalie Goldberg, *Wild Mind* (New York, NY: Bantam, 1990).

2. Linda Frazer Fleming, *Releasing Arthritis* (Falls Church, VA: LF Publishing, 1990).

# 5 Creating a Healing Environment

*Yes, you can fly! But your cocoon will have to go.*

When a situation becomes difficult, when we feel lost, alone, or are diagnosed with an illness, we are faced with two paths, and it isn't immediately obvious which of these we'll walk. Both paths start out in hope, but rarely do we change without effort and struggle.

We may experience many setbacks in our journey to emotional, physical, and spiritual health because healing involves complex changes on every level of our being. Along the way, within our own subterranean spiritual catacombs, we evaluate the cost of staying in physical life, working to heal, as well as the cost of leaving the Earth. No one chooses consciously to die or stay sick. This means we don't make that life choice at the personality level. Spiritual crisis teaches us to dig and dig and dig to touch the spiritual levels of our core, where we do consider the larger issues of our existence.

## The Power of Choice in Healing

I've had many clients, and some of them have changed dramatically and moved into more fulfilling lives while others have struggled and seemingly never found the spiritual energy to cause their lives to really work well. As someone involved intimately in people's life-and-death struggles, I've found that a person can benefit from considering the meaning of his or her own death or change in consciousness in order to come to terms with the meaning of his or her life. The "no-man's land" between the two extremes of life and transition is a place without power or support for our healing. Lasting healing comes from facing our lives and our death and deciding in which camp we want to place our energy. No matter the drugs or surgeries or extravagant means modern technology employs to keep us alive, it is our spirit that awakens our own deepest loving energy to help us make this shift toward physical life or away from it.

A true-life story comes to mind of a nine-year-old boy who discovered he had an inoperable tumor at the base of his skull. In the book, *Why Me?* Garrett Porter and Patricia Norris tell Garrett's story of healing. Garrett remembers the night he came to terms with his own death as the point at which he truly began to embrace life. He recounts that he had called his dad into his room and asked him to sit down on the side of his bed. He asked his dad if he was going to die! His father responded that this was a possibility. Garrett remembers staying awake all night, and as the first rays of dawn began to break, he said to himself, "I am going to live." Through those hours of the night he reviewed his options and his future and drifted somewhere beyond himself to consider his monumental choice. Beneath the personality level, deep within him, the power of his spirit came forth into his life and activated his own power, his will power to live. He chose to live, and in fact he did.

The father's response was especially significant because it is unimaginably difficult to tell your child that he or she might die. We want to rush in to protect the one we love, telling the person that everything will be all right—we will make it right, by the force of our diligence, determination, and sheer power of will. But, of course, we can't make it right. Only the child can look into him- or herself and find and tap the eternal spirit. Garrett's father offered the best he had, which was an honest answer. Actually, I've found that when we are able to be honest in response to the questions of those who are sick or hurting, we give others the power of choice, and that this is the way to awaken their own will power. When we deprive a person of this choice, disease can creep up and overtake a person's physical presence without the person's ever having a chance to rally his or her spirit.

## Awakening the Body's Natural Healing Energy

Our emotions help us understand and appreciate the God-force because they help us find the God within ourselves. Learning to see Love in the Divine presence requires knowing that Love lives inside us. We discover that this is as true today as it was in the time of Jesus and before. The Sacred lives in all of us, and today our opportunity is to accentuate these qualities in ourselves, in those people close to us, and in those whom our lives touch only occasionally.

We can heal whether we need to recover from a life-threatening illness, an emotional breakdown, or the severe loss of a partner or family member. What is required, though, is to awaken the body's natural healing energies to combat the negative and painful aspects of our situation. When that positive energy is activated, the old parts of our individual personality that cooperated with disease or that devalued or diminished our worth will wither. In other words, the physical body can be revitalized and encouraged when its own energy and the emotional energy of personal worth and spiritual love merge inside.

When it is others who need to heal, as much as we want to help those people we love we can only create a healing environment for them. The persons we love must themselves cause the essential inner shift toward Love and interaction with the God-force if they are to stay in physical life or experience substantial positive change.

## Choosing Your Own Team of Healers

I use the word *healer* to include all those in traditional or complementary medicine, those offering any sort of therapy or psychological counseling, and those in the ministry or spiritual counseling. This all-inclusive definition recognizes the fact that each of us is a healer, actually or potentially. Healing comes naturally to all of us, even though we are the most comfortable in interacting with others in certain specific ways.

The foundation for the entire medical community is the Hippocratic oath, the symbol of two snakes woven together as a shield. Physicians take this oath before being allowed to work with patients. This symbol speaks to the compassion, trust, and wisdom assumed by those who would work with others toward healing. This is the level of insight and care that you want in those who work with you. Assume that this is their motivation, and if you discover that it is absent, make other choices.

All too often we feel we must play games, keeping our more traditional healing helpers, physicians, therapists, and-ministers from interacting with those who love us or espouse amore all-encompassing and holistic approach to healing. Recognize that our healing progress is less effective when we keep separated those who love and wish us well.

## Assembling Your Personal Healing Wheel

One night, while I was working on a client, she began to talk about the nature of being sick and of having struggled with cancer through recurrence after recurrence. She said, "I'm tired of things that I have to do. My entire life has been made up of things that needed to be done to reach this or that goal. I want to experience just being with myself and others in a loving way. I'm so hungry to be part of a loving community of people. I just want to sit and absorb love, and I know if I could do this I'd get better."

It's time to recognize that we need others, that "loving community of people," to facilitate our individual healing, especially when we are struggling with severe pain or a debilitating illness or loss. One of the most effective support systems that I've used with clients is the healing wheel.

If you are the person in need of healing, picture in your mind the image of a wheel in which the members of your team of healers and helpers are the spokes of the wheel. Then place yourself at the center or hub. Symbolically and actually, you've created a vehicle for achieving wholeness, the goal of healing. It doesn't matter whether the members of your team come from traditional or complementary medical practices or are family or close friends. What does matter is that they care about you, and you trust them.

People have interesting responses to being instructed to place themselves in the center of their own healing wheel. Women especially often ask if that isn't being selfish and self-centered. These responses point up the degree to which we've all buried our own appreciation of our unique value. For too long, we've absorbed the message that to talk about ourselves or our accomplishments is an undesirable thing: it's selfish, self-centered, and conceited. We've naturally generalized this message to mean that, since we aren't to talk about our worth, we obviously aren't supposed to have any. When I suggest that people are to make their needs known to others, to stop hiding and to come forward with their own goodness, value, and worth, they feel intimidated, as if doing this were wrong. To affirm our inner value we need to express our worth in conversation.

When we are healing we need to be around positive, loving people. The spokes of your healing wheel should be people who are unafraid to give because they understand that we all give and receive at different times in our lives and around different issues. We need other people. No one can heal in a vacuum.

The last part of your healing wheel is your healing coach, an individual who will support and guide you at the center.

## Selecting Your Healing Coach

A person who lives nearby and who sincerely cares about helping you heal can assume the role of healing coach. This person plays a special part in your work to heal and recover by encouraging the growth of spiritual energy. He or she needs no particular medical background but is someone you feel comfortable with in talking about the discouraging parts of your journey as well as the positive and affirming ones. This person should be comfortable placing his or her hands on you (on top of your clothes) to awaken the energy of your body. Later on in the book, we will be talking about using this method of helping you heal.

The healing coach is the person you can call late at night or early in the morning, the one from whom you know you'll receive a large dose of emotional and spiritual aid. People often choose for their healing coach a partner or spouse, or a close friend or a therapist, or a person they have done body work with, such as Reiki, acupuncture, acupressure, polarity, or massage. It can be any person you trust and feel good about being with, and who helps you make choices for your treatment and will guide acquaintances and friends in meeting your needs.

Your healing coach might go with you to medical appointments to be sure that the questions you are concerned about get answered. Your healing coach is the one whom you are comfortable talking to, or whose shoulder you can cry on, or whose support you can ask for in between the major doctor appointments and the time when the professionals in your life are not reachable. This is a key person, and both you and your healing coach enter a unique and poignant relationship in exploring the dynamics of spiritual energy and potential healing. This work with your healing coach will be instrumental in helping you both grow emotionally and spiritually.

Sometimes people in need of healing help can't think of a person who fits the role of healing coach. I've found that if we accept that this person will find us, then we can

go about creating our healing wheels anyway, and magically, the right person joins us enroute. Our job is to acknowledge the need for this person and then to turn that need
over to the Universe, knowing that others will be drawn to
us by the power of our intention.

## The Power of Your Healing Wheel

Choosing and acknowledging those we want to work with
us as part of our healing wheels gives us great inner power.
We become more effective in decision-making. We feel we
have the right and obligation to oversee what is happening
to us, to ask solid questions from our caregivers, and to
expect quality and meaningful exchange and help.

An important benefit from the healing wheel is that
others can participate with us in ways that allow them to
honor their own vision and skills. We often feel that we are
always on the receiving end—that others always tell us
what we've done wrong but never acknowledge our
strengths and skills. Sometimes we need to be the one giving rather than receiving the Love. When we are in need of
help we obviously need the attention of others, but as we
get better and more aligned with our own wholeness ourselves, we can then offer caring attention to others.

I've found that some friends and family members find it
meaningful to join their own prayers or meditations directly
to the person working to heal. And so people have used
specific affirmations to support their own inner work and to
benefit those they love. The more people you have holding
you in their prayers and meditations, the stronger the energy you can draw toward your own healing. Even repeating
the same phrase and intention increases energy. An example might be, "I_____(the person sending healing energy)

offer loving thoughts and abundant health and well-being to
_____(the name of the person needing  healing)."

If you need to heal through loss or disease, ask special
friends and family to participate in your healing wheel.
This gives you a chance to quietly assume your role as the
one making appropriate choices on your own behalf.  Your
request also tells your friends that this is a relationship and
an experience that you take seriously, as an opportunity for
life healing, and so there is a good chance they will do the
same.  The responsibilities for this work require that your
friends and team meet your needs in ways that fit your
needs.  This may mean gathering your family and friends
together to discuss parts of your care, or to pray together, or
to discuss spiritual subjects in books relevant to your healing.  This healing wheel is your mini-support group, and it
really works to help you feel stable and aware during times
that can be personally stressful.

As we assume responsibility for our healing wheels and
become part of the healing wheel of others, we discovers
that words alone are often unable to convey our Love and
desire to have others help us or to help others.  We are all
part of a community of people, and our balance and full
attention and participation is required if we hope to shift
the course of personal or planetary disease to health and
well-being.

# 6 The Role of the Healing Coach

*Healing is natural, and so is helping others who are in pain.*

As the diatribe over national health care continues, funding for wellness programs dries up, home health-care services are slashed, and community resources are overtaxed, we find ourselves at the edge of an enormous crevasse. We know something must be done, and yet we continue to wait for others to release the dollars, to formulate the programs to provide relief. While we are certainly addressing significant health-care questions to rescue ourselves and those we love, we still continue to look to the old models of healing and health-related services. It's time to acknowledge that another approach to healing and health care is emerging and that it arises authentically from our connection to family, friends, and community.

We have become used to thinking of healing in terms of physicians, nurses, and related health-care practitioners.

We also now recognize the plethora of holistic physicians, body-workers, and counselors guiding us in approaches to wellness that pay attention to mind and spirit as well as to body. And yet, if someone in our family has cancer, if a friend is facing unemployment, if an acquaintance is chronically sick, we are all too aware that their needs are not being adequately met even by the legions of people in these established roles.

Medical science has continued to pour millions of dollars into technological advances that help some but that are moving physicians too far away from their patients. Medicine has become a business, with medical practitioners and nurses caught squarely in the middle. While it may seen impractical to return to the age of house calls, the position of "family doctor" who is also a friend has nevertheless been vacated and needs to be filled. We've abdicated our closeness with those in trouble in favor of more efficient, but not necessarily better, ways of helping them.

When we are in trouble or hurting, we don't want a machine or a sterile environment, we want Love, attention, community, and care of our needs by a real person who has time for us. We need help based on Love and a willingness to participate in our lives. This is the role of what I call the healing coach. The healing coach assumes not the scientific role of the physician but the compassionate and supportive role of the "family doctor."

A healing coach offers a holistic approach at the grassroots level that helps people heal their lives. We don't need red tape, limitations, stipulations, and bureaucratic stumbling blocks when we or our loved ones are hurting and need help and attention. Until we accept our own capacity to nurture and help those close to us heal, we will be unable to change the system. Until we believe that we have the time if we take the time. Until we acknowledge that we are all part of a community, and that together we can effectively and meaningful meet each other's needs.

## We Cannot Heal Alone

In our busy lives, we've assumed that our time could best be spent earning more money to pay for the services we need. Perhaps we need to consider our caretaking roles as family, friends, and community members as offering more to those we love than only sending them to experts.

When we face life-threatening illness, serious loss, or momentous change, we are headed for a period without the energy or perspective to meet all our own needs and make all our own decisions. We cannot heal alone. We need a healing coach to help us choose what we want and need. We need someone to be available to us in between our major medical appointments or treatments—someone who cares, is a good listener, and has a capacity to love. We need someone who can help us get our practical needs met. And we need someone who is comfortable touching us.

## The Qualities of a Good Healing Coach

This capacity to love is the single most important ingredient in being a healing coach because it is the emotional energy of Love that can be used in simple massage, stroking, holding, and hands-on attention to best facilitate healing. Many times we feel squeamish about touching someone because we are afraid we may hurt that person or that he or she won't like it. Being touched is the most important contact we have with each other, and most people who are sick or feeling lost or lonely suffer most from a lack of physical

touching.  Physical touching with a basic level of understanding of the nature of the body's energy reduces pain
and facilitates the body's natural healing processes.

Being a healing coach requires our developing a basic
understanding of the interconnection between the body,
mind, and spirit.  The aspects to being a healing coach that
I use and encourage in my work with others include:

- learning simple massage and energy balancing to
  soothe,  relax, and encourage physical healing;

- teaching holistic thinking to reassure the mind;

- using Love and our personal attention to draw forth
  feelings of self-worth; and

- sharing and participating in prayer, meditation,
  and/or quiet times to witness the process of spiritual
  growth.

## Your Job Is to Encourage the Search for
## Spiritual Imbalances

In our western culture, we are not set up to meet people's
needs in a holistic way.  We are set up to address separate
symptoms or imbalances, but the ailing person has a difficult time assimilating various paths to healing into one com-
prehensive package.  We also tend to accentuate the importance of physical and emotional change without adequately
addressing spiritual change.  From my work and observa-
tions I know that all meaningful change begins on the
deepest spiritual levels and gradually works its way outward
into our emotions and physical bodies.

Spiritual change consists of re-evaluating our relationship with the God-force in order to find some reason for
our suffering and to rediscover our capacity to love our-

selves enough to make the choices to ensure for ourselves a meaningful future. Without a sense of alignment with the God-force, people feel disempowered and disconnected from their purposes. When healing has no grounding in the spiritual, the body and emotions only "go through the motions" of healing, and no significant energy is activated on an internal level. When people are in the throes of physical disease, are losing energy, are afraid they may die, are unsure of the treatment choices they've made or need to make, their focus has drifted to the disease rather than to the basic spiritual imbalance that has allowed the disease to enter the body. As healing coach we can help our friend or client by encouraging a spiritual search to right old imbalances.

## Pointing the Way to a Future

As healing coach, part of your work is to expand your loved one's perspective to include a meaningful future. What does the person want to do with his or her life? What stands in the way for the person to have a future, and if he or she heals, what painful emotional situation will need to be faced? Sometimes it seems easier to die.

A client told me of his own life-or-death dilemma, one that is characteristic of many people. He was trying to decide whether to have chemotherapy and radical surgery to address the cancer in his body. As we expanded the focus of our discussion from the depressing array of choices for traditional cancer treatment and began to talk about his future, he recognized the point of real conflict in his life, the conflict that was impinging on his efforts to heal. He realized that if he were to heal he would probably need to leave his wife, because he had known for a long time that she didn't share his value system and that their relationship wasn't working.

When our focus is placed on the future we hope to create for ourselves, those elements that hinder this growth fall out into our laps to be dealt with. They also fall into the lap of the healing coach to gently share what is felt.

Our suffering brings us a new perspective. It shows us we are required to lean in a direction that honors our own beliefs and to speak out in ways that heal the crippled, old emotions we've lived with and that have made us sick. A client recounts the dream she had of her future. She was standing on a path, and a huge pile of boulders lay in front of her. She could just barely make out the path on the other side of the boulders, and it was light and beautiful. She knew her journey was to get over those seemingly insurmountable rocks to reach the other side. The next night the same dream reappeared, and she found herself actually climbing the rocks. She had begun her healing journey and was claiming a different future.

## Understanding the Needs of Your Friend/Client

One of the greatest sources of confusion and pain to a person mired in spiritual crisis is the sense of aloneness it brings. In choosing an approach to healing, we find many demands made on our time, and we are required to address many levels of healing. We have many new appointments, many changes in our diet, hygiene, attitudes, and spiritual work. Yet the need for personal contact and loving community remains constant.

A client summed it up when she said, "I feel so shut off from people. I long to have meaningful bonds with people, but I'm usually too tired by the time I do all the things I'm suppose to do in my healing programs. And when I am with people in small groups, I don't know what to say to adequately express my feelings. Others who are healthy don't seem to have my needs. I want to reach out and hold on to these bonds with people. I just don't know the words to use and why I'm feeling so starved for love. It's very discouraging."

As a person in need of healing, you want to be loved and nurtured without having to "do" anything to earn or deserve it. As a healing coach, you can gently yet persistently be available to work and help in whatever ways are desirable and beneficial to your healing friend. You are intent upon expanding positive loving energy in your friend's life, and to do this you accept a deeper level of your own intuitive guidance.

## The Gifts You Receive

When you give your Love in the form of service to others, you receive something quite precious in return: the confirmation of your own life purpose.

You may have wanted to understand your life purpose but were unsure where to begin to search for it. You may have been asking, "What does my life mean?" "What can I do to help?" "In what way am I to use my skill and abilities?" You look for something tangible that will be recognizable as your purpose. When you are actually doing things to help as opposed to wondering what things you should be doing, your purpose taps you on the shoulder. One day you observe yourself in action and realize that this thing that you are doing or participating in to help feels so right and wonderful because it is what you are supposed to be doing. Your purpose is so close to us that you use it continually without recognizing it. The desire to be of service, as a global energy, is awakening in your soul because it is the basis for building a culture based on holism and mutual prosperity.

The experience of being someone's healing coach may open your own doorway to your purpose. Often, acting as if you are presently using the part of your purpose you know brings additional aspects into view.

The archetype of healer is emerging as the dominant blueprint of our time. If you are drawn to helping another person, consider that you may be feeling the impact of this pattern of "healer" because becoming a healer may be your purpose.

We tend to confuse our purpose with the ways we earn a living. These two paths ideally come together into one, but at the beginning this is not necessarily so. When we first recognize something we love doing, like helping another person by listening, by laying our hands on the person in a loving way, we may still be earning a living in a way that is seemingly unrelated. If we are to journey further down the road of healer, then a way to support ourselves will emerge all by itself, with little help from us. A prayer in our hearts that says, "Let me be of service to the God-force in the most appropriate way, and let me see my avenue of service so clearly that I can't miss it" may be the simple affirmation sufficient to open doorways to us.

We need to be mentally and emotionally prepared to act and learn at the same time. We don't even need to know what the next day will bring for our purposes to be drawn to us. I've found that "being available to daily guidance" is the most important spiritual lesson I've ever learned. I ask before making choices, "Does this feel right?" "Am I receiving a sense of being supported in this decision?" "Are the pieces of this plan coming together easily, or am I struggling to make it work?" Listening for the energy of our spirits that supports our actions is an essential skill for making choices that support our purposes and help create our desired future.

# You Are the Instrument of Healing, Not the Healing Force

Energy is the force at the basis of all life, and when we accept that it is fluid rather than rigid, we experience its power. When we have overstepped and outdistanced the flow of energy within us, we feel a hollowness—a lack of inner support for our actions. At such times we need to back up in our actions and initiatives to the place where we again feel a sense of the flow of alive energy. Feeling without energy happens in working with others when, for the best reasons, we assume we know what someone else needs, and we've rushed prematurely toward assumed conclusions. We can become so busy asserting our wisdom, knowledge, and certainties that we forget to listen.

Healing is a profound exchange between two people of loving energy that activates the God-force within each soul. You, the healing coach, are also meant to gain from this exchange, though in a way that prevents you from depleting your own energy. If you are exhausted rather than exhilarated after working on a person, it means you've been drawing too much from your own energy reserves and not enough from the Universe's. As a healing coach, you are merely a conduit for eternal and totally essential loving energy that is meant to be absorbed into the body of the person on whom you are working. Because some energy demand is made on your own body, physically and emotionally, you need to be healthy to work on others so that taking away energy doesn't impair your own health.

## Learning to Love More Completely

We can never appreciate fully what another person feels at times of greatest challenge. The best we can do is to resist forming opinions or judgements. We can be useful by bringing our love to bear and being present and responsive in ways that seem appropriate. Spiritual work begins when the shock has worn off and the person begins to face what is required to mend or adjust his or her situation.

Whether we are in the role of a healing coach or dealing with our own crisis, we frequently need many inner forays into our spiritual midst. Most of us have little experience understanding our lives in terms of universal law. We find it extremely difficult to learn that our spiritual systems are directing our lives when all the time we thought our mental systems were. At stressful times, our mental and spiritual systems are at war, each pulling in the opposite direction. We feel angry, anything but loving. Yet inside, we are being hollowed out in order to experience expansive feelings that are made possible by our loss and pain. When we grieve for those we love, we awaken an even deeper capacity to love. Life requires us to gain insight into Divine awareness. We learn to love so that we can use the energy of Love with others. Sometimes it is through the prospect of losing those we love most that we truly gain the capacity to love more completely.

## Some Final Advice

Spiritual work sounds good and makes sense, yet we still expect that when we find the magic button, push the right lever, we'll get better immediately. We forget that the process of spiritual change is ongoing, not merely a goal to be reached when our mission has been accomplished.

With this understanding we are better prepared to serve in healing work. So remember to begin with a loving heart and an open mind, resolved to merely be present to help in whatever way you feel is right. Even if a disease seems to be getting worse in the person you're helping, accept that you both have whatever time is required to chart your course toward healing, whether that means staying in or leaving physical life. Your moments together, including those pithy as well as protracted conversations, will be healing for your friend and you. Healing happens not according to any set schedule but when timing is in place. Let the rate of your healing work be dictated by your friend or client.

I'm assuming that because you are reading this book you have some basis of interest in the field of spirituality. If you are new to this field yourself, then admit this openly to the other person, at the same time expressing your desire for the two of you to learn together.

When you work with others, it's always a question of who gets the most from the shared time. I like to begin to work with others by assuming that I am the student and they are the teachers. The person you're helping is having the experience; your work is to effectively mirror and complement the inner work that the person is initiating. Healing comes as we absorb Love for ourselves and others. Healing is always possible but becomes a reality when we awaken the energy of Love from ourselves and the God-force and then give it freedom to find its mark within the heart of another.

# 7 Energy: The Invisible Life Force

*To conceive of life as it truly is, you must leave the
state of physical reality and venture into the world
of spiritual energy.*

In healing, energy is the key to the invisible world. Energy
moves us toward increased understanding of the nature of
our stay here on the Earth. It is drawn into our systems in a
number of ways but most significantly through the top of
the head, through the heart, or through the solar plexus.
This means we draw energy into ourselves and generate
our own supply of positive energy as we are able to accept
our own self-worth, to live in a loving way, and to listen
and work with the needs of our bodies and their wisdom.

Healing our own lives and helping others heal involves
synthesizing the energies of our bodies, minds, and spirits.
If we concentrate on learning the ways in which we create
energy, if we are able to generate our own supply of energy
to accentuate what we absorb, and if we understand the

ways in which energy drains away from us, we are on our way to creating health. We can increase our ability to hold energy in our bodies by clearing the energy channels that can be blocked with dysfunctional emotional responses. We also need to increase our capacity to participate, through our spiritual study, in the honing of our relationship with the Divine. By engaging in this clearing process we improve our ability to sustain the energy of the God-force and to also draw from life the complementary loving energy to support us.

This means that as we understand energy, we appreciate our opportunity to change what has already come into being and influence what still remains in the possibility or probability state—that is, "in the ether."

## Interpreting Feedback from Your Emotions and Physical Senses

One way we experience our inner well-being is through our moods. While moods are not always accurate interpreters of our health, we nevertheless know when we feel positive and creative and appreciative of ourselves and others. At those times we can assume we are building positive energy. The opposite is also true: when we are depressed, angry, and upset with ourselves, we slow down the energy assimilation in our bodies and our total energy field.

A deeper and more accurate assessment of our energy well-being comes from sensing whether we are working "on purpose" with our lives or groping for the missing piece. We may feel sad but fail to understand the source of our sadness. We may feel disconnected from life and lonely even though we may have a partner or family living with us. We may feel incomplete in some significant way. Such feelings alert us to internal imbalances and lack of energy resources. Awareness and subsequent healing of such imbalances and lacks is essential for continued health.

Feedback from our physical senses allows us to experience our environment. For better or worse we can see, taste, smell, feel, and hear our world. Our senses give us crucial information so that we can function effectively and gain pleasurable feedback from the world around us. In our hurry-up lives, however, we are forced to take too little time to fully assimilate, to digest, our perceptions of people, our past experiences, and life in general. We speed toward our tomorrows without fully processing our experiences of today.

While some of our life experiences are assimilated easily, others require more attention, and yet we swallow them half-digested. Feelings around loss often remain unprocessed. Fear of being abandoned, fear of being found valueless, remain within us, imprinting their messages upon our physical tissues. Gradually, our bodies break down from the sheer weight of these unprocessed messages. Processing loss effectively involves moving beneath the personality level to the inner plane of spirit where we find our true selves and our relationship to the God-force.

## The Three Levels of Life-force Energy

Life-force energy flows continually through our systems, and when part of our energy network breaks down we experience breakdown in our lives. In order to help ourselves or each other, we need to understand that even though the physical body may be sick or have a tumor or a degenerative condition, or the emotions may be flattened because of divorce or a death in the family, what is truly impaired is the flow of energy throughout our systems. We all have short-term impairments, but when our energy fields are diminished by long-standing disabilities, our health and well-being suffer noticeably. A lack of energy in our bodies means that we are unable to do those things we most want to do or to function in ways that are meaningful to us.

The energy of life-force is similar to a braid with many levels of energy entwined. Our health is the result of these energy currents weaving throughout our physical, emotional, and spiritual bodies. Each of these strands makes up a level of our energy field, or even sub-levels, or more finely defined levels of energy. Healer-author Barbara Brennan, in her book *Hands of Light*, describes the many levels of energy she sees clairvoyantly and the results she's had in healing a wide variety of diseases and disturbances.[1] Most people do not actually see these levels of energy, but they are there. The three most significant levels of energy are the etheric, the astral, and the spiritual.

1. The etheric energy level is the physical body's blueprint of perfection. I call this blueprint the "body wisdom" or "wise body."

2. The astral energy level is the sensing, feeling, and thinking aspect of our consciousness.

3. The spiritual energy level is the awakened soul and spiritual exchange with the God-force. This level specifically involves the six influences of Love that I've discussed in Chapter Three.

For a graphic presentation of these levels of energy, see Figure 2, "The Etheric, Astral, and Spiritual Energy Fields, Including the Six Spiritual Energy Influences of Love."

Each of these levels of energy—etheric, astral, and spiritual—is significant, because each is affected by everything we

## *Figure 2:*
## The Etheric, Astral, and Spiritual Energy Fields, Including the Six Spiritual Energy Influences of Love

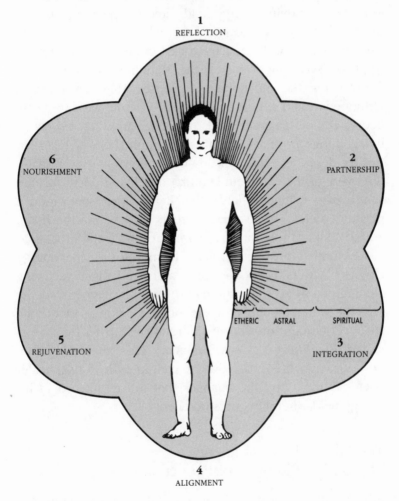

1
REFLECTION

6
NOURISHMENT

2
PARTNERSHIP

ETHERIC    ASTRAL    SPIRITUAL

5
REJUVENATION

3
INTEGRATION

4
ALIGNMENT

think, do, are, and profess to believe. When we seek to heal the body we must also establish a new relationship with each of these levels, because each level shifts and changes in relationship to new attitudes, insights, and experiences.

Physicians and scientific researchers have for many years been studying energy fields, and today energy and its uses in healing are receiving special attention. Scientists like Elmer Green, Ph.D., Director Emeritus of the Center for Applied Psychophysiology at the Menninger Foundation in Topeka, Kansas, and Robert O. Becker, M.D., Professor of Orthopedics and author of *The Body Electric*, have for years been studying magnetic fields of energy and the currents all living things produce that flow through these fields. Dr. Becker describes this work in "bio energy" as "the primary discovery of the twentieth century: that living organisms are sensitive to magnetic fields, that living organisms produce magnetic fields, that electric currents flow within the body, and that all of these things are a part of the living process."[2]

Scientists are also effectively monitoring the energy changes within the bodies of healers and those receiving healing energy to study the nature of both magnetic energy and the etheric energy of the body wisdom. One such study documenting energy in relationship to healing is called *Bio Energy: A Healing Art*. This interesting film describes the life and work of well-known Polish healer Mietek Wirkus and the changes that are monitored in his energy field when he works on clients.[3]

## The Etheric Level of Energy: The Body's Blueprint of Perfection

Etheric energy surrounds the physical body and holds the blueprint for perfect health. Placing our hands on a person and seeing ourselves as a channel for Universal Love helps the physical body rediscover its perfect health image. In order to heal, you are reacquainting your physical body with its own blueprint, or body wisdom. When you get sick, have pain, and experience disease, your body's relationship with its own perfection has been interrupted. In healing, the image of perfect health and functioning is again imparted to the cells, organs, and systems, and the body is therefore better able to function.

In whatever ways we relieve pain and distress within the body, we must never forget that drugs, medicine, or treatments of any kind only give us time to do the other inner work that is basic to maintaining our health. By reducing pain and tension, we haven't solved the problems, we've just pushed them out of sight temporarily. The spiritual challenge is to still seek the emotions that overloaded our physical circuits and the reasons we are lacking in the life-force energy that recharges our systems continually.

The physical body is like a fuse box. When we get sick or are in pain, the fuse blows, and the lights go out. While we can put in a new fuse, we still have to reconnect the physical body with the etheric energy, the body wisdom, in order to get the "new-fuse" response. When we awaken the energy of our spirits and the God-force in our lives, the lights go on, because we have re-set the circuit breaker.

Plants and animals, along with people, have etheric energy fields that hold the pattern of their own perfection. We can see this dramatically in a process called "sensitive crystallization," developed by Dr. Ehrenfried Pfeiffer, a colleague of the noted scientist and founder of Anthroposophy, Rudolf Steiner.[4] Etheric energy that surrounds the body is different from electromagnetic energy, for instance.

top of a magnet, the iron filings arrange themselves in such a way as to always form the positive and negative images of the magnetic field. If we put several drops of an extract from a living plant into a salt solution and then let the solution crystallize out, or dry up, we see something quite dramatically different. The crystals from the plant arrange themselves to give an image of the living substance studied!

This experiment is fascinating because it suggests that the invisible etheric energy of one piece of a living thing holds in its "memory" the perfect whole. This is exactly what we are discovering in working with the body wisdom, or blueprint of perfect health, that we each have as part of our own energy fields. When we are successful in awakening the body's ability to sense and re-accept its total wholeness and perfect health, physical symptoms disappear.

Increasing evidence also suggests that in addition to etheric energy, the body also requires overall balancing of its total electricity or electromagnetic fields. This total-body balancing is used in many complementary health approaches that focus on rebuilding a person's immune system in order to eliminate such imbalances as cancer, Alzheimer's syndrome, multiple sclerosis, and cystic fibrosis. Healing occurs when the body's systems recognize the changes that are required and set about making them. The study of the subtle energy bodies of all living things is, without doubt, the field of "new medicine" for the future.

## The Astral Level of Energy:
## The Emotional and Mental Bodies

People have come to understand astral energy as the energy seen in auras or the halos reported by early mystics and intuitives. The colors in a person's aura change continually and reflect a person's moods, health, emotional and mental well-being, and spiritual Love.

Our thoughts, beliefs, and attitudes, our psychological and emotional processing of information and feelings, are represented in this astral layer of energy. This energy is affected by all the input from a person's body, spirit, and living environment.

Positive words and feelings produce positive energy, and negative words and feelings drain energy, having a deleterious effect on the physical body and its state of emotional health and balance. Emotions, both positive and negative, affect the ways in which energy is able to regenerate and to move throughout the body. While specific emotions encourage our personal growth and physical healing, others impede this development. The way we feel when we think certain positive or negative thoughts, or the way we react when we're on the receiving end of certain emotions, gives us a good idea of their effect on the body and whether or not they are contributing to our body wisdom or perfect health. When we feel shamed, undervalued, or diminished, our body vitality withers. And when we feel honored, appreciated, and loved, our body wisdom is reinforced, and health is encouraged.

The following table lists emotions that we all feel from time to time, with their responses from the physical body.

*anger* — drains energy from the body, leaving it "energy-anemic"

*fear* — solidifies energy, immobilizing the physical body, distressing the emotions, and reducing the focus of spirit

*pain* — stalls energy, reducing the body's ability to metabolize food; reduces its capacity to regenerate cellular tissue *resentment* — slowly erodes energy, causing depression of all functions

*guilt* — slows energy movement among organs and systems, reducing the body's capability to mend and replace cells

*loss* — diminishes energy exchange among the three levels of life-force energy and makes it more difficult for the physical body to reflect perfection from the body wisdom

*compassion* — couples and uncouples complex energies so that they can be absorbed readily by the physical body

*love* — reinforces the body wisdom or etheric level of energy, specifically energizing the physical brain, heart tissues, and the immune system; is also a major factor in balancing the astral or thinking and feeling level of energy

*excitement* —releases bursts of energy that reinforce the endocrine system, revitalizing the fluids of the body

*reverence*—gives the spirit permission to direct the body wisdom, with specific regard to the defining of one's purpose and future effectiveness.

*acceptance*—enhances peacefulness within the body energies, allowing the spirit and God-force connection to become apparent

## The Spirit Level of Energy: Love and Spiritual Energy

Prayer, meditation, and quiet time in nature can either recharge our spirits, releasing joy for the blessing of our lives and Love for our courage in the challenges we face, or they can be perfunctory routines that leave us feeling empty and alone.

Spiritual energy comes from an assurance that the God-

even if we can't understand the
The greatest challenge to healing
his spark of universal life and to
forth in our lives to permeate
actions. Spiritual energy is the
ind has the six aspects of influ-
er: Reflection, Partnership, Inte-
tion, and Nourishment.

this life with the opportunity to
decide individually to put that
e Love, give Love, respond to
of Love if we hope to with-
ind individual spiritual crisis.
Planning to do it later doesn't
t done it before doesn't help.
d to others, builds essential

## NOTES

1. Barbara Brennan, *Hands of Light* (New York, NY: Bantam Books).

2. New World Media Alliance, *Bio Energy: A Healing Art* (Bethesda, MD: Wirkus Bioenergy Foundation).

3. *Ibid.*

4. Victor Bott, *Anthroposophical Medicine* (New York, NY: Thorsons Publishers, Inc.), p. 23.

# 8 Building Positive Emotional Energy From Self-Worth

*As we each heal the pain from our emotional losses we become an asset rather than a liability to those around us.*

For all the self-help books and articles written to encourage people in reclaiming their wholeness and personal power, we are still a culture in search of an inner identity. We hope to find our lives' meaning, yet rarely do we know where to look to find the treasure map with the pot of gold clearly marked. No quick answer realigns us with our self-worth or the Universe. We do this for ourselves, one step at a time, acknowledging our desire to participate fully in life. The only way toward finding our self-worth is, as a popular saying goes, the old fashioned way: we earn it.

Finding our own inner goodness, our self-worth, is essen-

tial to transcending the dark night of the soul of spiritual crisis. Awakening our emotional energy of self-worth moves us
closer to the energy of our spirits and our relationship with
the God-force. Healing requires a positive stream of energy
from our spirits, from our emotions and thoughts, and also
from the energy of our body wisdom—the etheric energy
level. In this chapter, I'll discuss the energy coming from our
emotions and specifically from our feelings around self-worth.

Our emotional (astral) energy and spiritual (spirit) energy are bonded into a life-sustaining relationship. These two
levels of energy each play a significant role in the total life-
force energy held within our bodies. Together, our emotions and our spirits give us the comfort of Love, joy, self-
acceptance, and self-approval. Finding our spirits and
unleashing this energy of Love is dependent upon our
assessing the emotional responses we use automatically and
upon weeding out responses that aren't growing from our
own self-worth. And so we'll begin to reach toward our
spiritual depth by first exploring our emotional responses to
our own spiritual crisis.

## Self-Esteem Is Different from Self-Worth

Self-esteem is different from self-worth. Self-esteem comes
from our actions or those of others affecting what we "do"
and what is done to us from the personality level. Self-
worth comes from our intentions and who we "are" from
our inner cores. Self-esteem is reinforced by others; self-
worth is reinforced by our own spirits that comment in positive ways about the quality of our actions. When we do
something for someone else, we feel something quite different than when someone does something for us.

When we are children, our emotional energy is like a

clean slate without others' marks upon it. As we grow up we internalize the messages and feedback from our world. This feedback is taken inside us and contributes to our security in seeking our self-worth. Or if our environment is negative and self-deprecating, we learn to hide our self-worth.

All the experiences that begin at the personality level through feedback and actions from others are interpreted by us and fed into our inner being. When we seek to heal, the positive or negative messages of others first reach our personality level and are internalized gradually, as messages that support or hinder our search for our self-worth. The more positive influences we have in our lives, obviously, the faster we become comfortable with remodelling our emotional responses.

We find our self-worth slowly and may continue for many years to question our value. As we become more confident in our self-worth, we find that we are not so easily shaken or full of self-blame when things go wrong in our lives. We tend to stick up for ourselves and believe in our assessments of people and circumstances; we don't immediately assume our own negligence or fault in a situation. We can't fool ourselves about self-worth. We know if we like who we are, if we feel we are living up to the expectations we've set for our lives. We can't pretend forever that we're fine when inside we feel hollow.

I like to think of self-worth as "inner goodness." Goodness is close to "Godness" and suggests that, emotionally, we can be in alignment with our own greatest and Universal good. The challenge in healing is not just having self-worth but in knowing that we have it and being able to draw strength from it at the conscious and easily-accessible personality level.

Our self-worth can be destroyed in less obvious ways

than by overt brutality or lack of attention. As we grow up we have trouble staying in touch with our self-worth because we learn from a variety of sources not to talk directly about our own needs or genuine accomplishments. This perception produces a deadly duality between the abilities and skills we know we have and our capacity to share and honor these with other people. Eventually, we forget that we have an inner goodness, and we spend our lives living with the fear that we possess no real value.

We humans require avenues of genuine expression through which we can say what is true for us and our lives. When we begin to find value in our thoughts, feelings, and actions, our own self-worth rises to the surface. We can honor our gifts as a reflection of the gifts bestowed upon us from the Universe.

Our own goodness is often so close to us, such a natural response, that we don't see it as our own unique contribution to life. We assume everyone's response is the same. Those qualities and traits that allow us to respond with warmth and compassion to another's needs, we dismiss. The people with the greatest goodness, holding the flame of hope for all of us, are those who are frequently the most blind to their own worth.

## The Story of Ruth

I'm reminded of a woman I met on the plane while traveling to California. Ruth's husband had died many years before, and she was on her way to visit her son and his wife and their new baby. As we talked about her life and mine, the issue of self-worth and personal value came up. She told me she'd never felt she had any real sense of worth or that she'd contributed very much to the world.

Yet the following story she related to me epitomizes the degree to which we overlook our own goodness. Because our good deeds are almost never accompanied by fanfare or broad recognition but are performed from a deep sacred place, we often fail to ascribe them to our self-worth.

Ruth lives in a sprawling big-city suburb. One day she was on her way to the grocery story when she passed a family standing on the street corner. The man held a sign indicating that he would work in exchange for food—that his wife and two children were hungry. All the way to the store Ruth thought about this family and the things this family might want and need. On her way home she drove back through the city to the corner where she had seen them standing. They were still there. She parked the car at the side of the road and walked up to the father. She asked him if he would be willing to accept the groceries—she had no work to offer. In stunned silence and with tears in his eyes he reached out for the groceries.

What touched me more than Ruth's generosity in buying the groceries was her concern for maintaining the man's dignity. Her attention was not on her own act of charity but on the feelings of her fellow human beings who needed help.

In Ruth's case she lived with the belief that she had no self-worth and was of no value to anyone. It didn't occur to her that the story she had recounted to me had any connection with self-worth. Like many others, Ruth had the gift of reaching out and helping others. Yet she lacked a sense of her own self-worth and felt diminished as a person.

## Finding Your Own Self-Worth

Without a strong and accurate sense of our own self-worth, we stay forever an arm's distance from the power and essential emotional energy required for healing. I once asked a woman who was in the process of redefining her life, and obviously undergoing spiritual crisis, what she felt was her own self-worth. She replied, "I have no idea. If I knew that I'd be able to heal."

An easy way to identify your self-worth is to observe it in motion as acts of service or helping. Think back over the last several months and remember circumstances in which you liked the ways you acted. They could include conversations you entered into or initiated or ways you effectively handled different home or work situations, all of which had positive outcomes. What did you do and what did you say that felt positive and appreciated? When you've answered these questions, you'll have loosely defined your own goodness—your self-worth.

## Validating Your Self-Worth

Here's an exercise that I've used successfully to help individuals identify and validate their own self-worth. As you think about your self-worth, take the time to write out a brief account of a scenario in which you found your self-worth. Then reduce the paragraph to a simple thought or a few sentences. Acknowledging your self-worth in writing holds twice as much power as merely recalling your story in your head. If you have trouble convincing yourself to take the time to do this simple exercise, recognize and honor the process that we go through to search through our inner feelings and experiences to find our truth. Validating your own self-worth is an essential element to healing. And in healing you are learning to make room for your more deeply-held beliefs, feelings, and emotional responses so that they can surface in your awareness. As you take the time to do this exercise, you open other doors through which your emotional energy can work for your healing and recovery. Because we can also learn from the ways others have identified their self-worth, I've included a number of examples.

### Joyce's Story

"My father was very ill, and the last time I went to visit him before he died I felt closer to him than ever before. I helped him talk through some of his fear and anxiety. I was calm and able to be practical at the same time. I helped him direct his thinking toward solutions that he obviously found meaningful and important."

*Joyce stated her self-worth this way:*
"I am able to give support and comfort to people in severe distress by helping them make essential choices and decisions."

### John's Story

"I volunteer in a nursing home, and most of the people there are all alone. No one comes to visit them, and even though most of the people don't make much sense, I read to them, tell them stories or jokes, or just listen. I know it helps them, even though they don't say so."

*John stated his self-worth this way:*
"I can make people feel better. It shrinks my own problems when I extend my focus to others in need."

### Melody's Story

"I teach at a progressive school that values personal balance and spiritual awareness as well as academic achievement. When young children have trouble adjusting to the school, and when the parents and members of the teaching staff are all trying to express their feelings about a particular child's situation, I'm able to help everyone feel acknowledged by conveying both enthusiasm and love."

*Melody stated her self-worth this way:*
"I use loving assertiveness on behalf of what I believe."

## Joan's Story

"A friend was in the hospital and was probably going to die very soon. I talked to her in a way that helped her look for the 'light' and not to be afraid. I told her that I knew she was getting ready to leave the Earth and spoke of how much she had meant to me. I reassured her of the meaningful and loving things she had done. I helped her die peacefully."

*Joan stated her self-worth this way:*
"I can accept and acknowledge other people's truth."

Recognizing our self-worth reminds me of the story of the three blind brothers, each attempting to explain the nature of an elephant. The first brother touched the tail, the second held the trunk, and the third brother felt a foot. Each brother had a valid description of the nature of an elephant based on his knowledge of it (the trunk, the tail or the foot), and yet the descriptions were very different.

Each time we encounter our self-worth it may seem different; yet the core aspect of our worth is always present in every situation where we seek to help or be of service. As soon as we become comfortable accepting our intentions and actions as positive and important for us and others, we allow the power and energy of our self-worth to play an increasingly important role in our lives. This emergence of our self-worth allows us to be compassionate, caring, giving, accepting, and also assertive. Those who exhibit the opposite qualities, insisting that we recognize their worth, show us that they are still searching for their value. True self-worth is recognized by others without our need to paint it out. If we have to tell others to honor, respect, and admire us, we are not yet there.

## Honesty in Relationships

Be honest about what you think and feel in your relationship with others. Ambiguous and poorly-defined relationships allow us to feel we have no self-worth. We often accept undefined and incomplete conversations and interactions with our partners, bosses, children, friends, and parents because we're afraid to hear what they really think about us. We often fear that we have no real value, so it's safer not to push for clarity.

People go to great extremes to maintain this secret. They will walk away from partners, long-standing friendships, careers, and even God in order to keep from having their fear confirmed. Like shining the light into a dark room, when we seek clarity in the intent of our actions we are telling others that we know we are of value, and so we want to know what they think and feel. We want our partners, bosses, lovers, even the God-force to speak directly to us about their purpose and intention because we are no longer afraid to hear the opinions of others. We know that we have purpose and intention.

Many times we seem unable to create the external world we want. We never seem to find the right job or the partner who meets our needs. A woman told me the story of her disastrous sixteen months in a job that had caused her great emotional pain and that eventually resulted in her getting seriously ill with a systemic neurological disease. She had found a career situation that promised great personal and professional success, but once hired, she felt let down by those who seemed to be friends and especially by her boss, whom she had assumed would be her mentor. So she left without telling anyone the way she felt and without sharing her perception of the situation.

Most people have a penchant for allowing fuzzy and ill-defined situations to exist in their relationships. Another client shared with me her feeling that all her life she'd chosen undefined relationships. She remembered early experiences when her parents would tell her how special she was because she had been adopted. She recounted feeling unworthy of these loving thoughts. Since she never told her parents what she really felt, she went on living with her ambivalence. Years later, she was still living with undefined relationships. Even in her professional relationships, when pressed for specific insight into her decisions or motives, she left a position rather than face her fear: that she had no real value. Rather than initiating a focussed discussion with co-workers, she chose to simply leave without closure or clarity. For marriage, she chose a man with similar fears, so they talked around issues without saying what they really meant. As she and I spoke, we realized the enormous implications for her life of not being honest about her true thoughts and feelings in her relationships with others.

If these two cases sound familiar, then consider that healing a lack of self-worth employs the same principle as skidding into a slide on an icy road. We are told to turn the steering wheel into the slide rather than in the opposite direction, the way that feels more normal. Likewise, we can learn to respond to upsetting and personally uncomfortable situations in our jobs and relationships by choosing actions that go contrary to the fearful responses, ones that seem the opposite of normal responses and yet deal directly with our feelings. Ask questions, seek confirmation, participate. Rather than waiting for life and people to disappoint us, we can seek clarity around relationship issues and initiate actions of our own. Either way, when we begin to initiate actions to clarify fuzzy situations, we are building the energy of self-worth. And when we are more willing and able to "take a chance" with asking people to be clear with us, we'll no longer be as afraid of what others will tell us. Whether positive or negative, flattering or distressing, we'll be able to deal effectively with the situation without our self-worth fears clouding our best judgement.

## The "Second Opinion" Emotions of Self-Worth

Before acting, allow your "second-opinion" emotional responses to shape your perspectives. The more you think and act in accord with your self-worth, the greater its energy and presence in your life and the better and more useful you feel to yourself and others. When you accept your self-worth, you create a mental resiliency that leaves "flex room" in your relationships. You don't always have to be right, you don't require others to always compliment you, you can make mistakes without being emotionally undone. You can roll more easily with the situations that life offers you and learn from them because your image of yourself is based on self-worth and not on illusion or fear.

We now know that we always have two perspectives from which to act. One reflects our fears and experiences that live at the personality level. The other perspective comes from deep within us, one that says that there is always a positive learning opportunity if we seek to discover it. So rather than listen to the feelings that are often the first that come to us in response to distress and that live only at the personality level, we need to learn to wait for a "second opinion." It is this second set of feelings that comes from our self-worth.

Before you decide that a person means to hurt you, that someone's intentions are negative, that others are in some way taking away from you or your family or your future, wait for the "second-opinion" emotions of your self-worth to click in. Wait, pause, hesitate, take the time necessary to allow these second-opinion emotional responses to rise up to show you a view of other people from a place of inner power and confidence. When you do this you benefit from the energy you are creating from your self-worth. You can thus respond in a way that is healing and empowered.

Acting in accord with our self-worth furthers our contribution to the planet and certainly to those close to us. Every time we self-select out those first emotions, the ones that are often fearful responses to feeling a lack of self-worth, and instead act from emotions motivated by self-worth, we give ourselves a tremendous gift. We come to experience real joy and inner peace. And as we adopt these new empowered ways of acting, we experience the flow of emotional energy into our bodies. The energy drawn from our own goodness allows our second-opinion responses to shape our perspectives before we act and thus creates a different outcome.

In striving to build our lives and our communities based on the energy of Love, we do well to remember that Love of self, Love of our Divine essence, is the core of self-worth. When we can identify our own goodness and put it to work, the negative becomes positive, the possible becomes actual, and our lives are filled with greater meaning and purpose.

# 9 Guardian Emotions Are Not Your Friends

*It is important to continually realize that you are in a position of taking back your life.*

Most of us over the years have used many kinds of responses to cover up our feelings of low self-worth. They all came from the ways we tried to get and keep the Love we needed. Sometimes we had to disown what we knew was true in order to keep from invalidating our parents—we needed to believe that they were right and that they loved us. Often we tried to deserve the Love that was so essential to us. We worked harder and harder to be good enough, to be perfect, to fit what others needed and wanted in order to be loved. We became experts at defusing the emotional bombs of anger, guilt, fear, and perhaps even physical abuse from dysfunctional parents or family members in order to get the Love that we still needed from them.

In our lives at present, we use the very same means of molding ourselves to fit the needs and expectations of others to get and keep the Love we need. The problem with this approach to life is that it causes us to recreate over and over again the very same painful scenarios from our past. We are sure that Love comes only in the strained and warped ways that we've experienced it from our past, so unconsciously we choose relationships and experiences that continually create the circumstances that most closely approximate our old familiar molds.

Of course, we're blind to the ways we contort ourselves and our lives to fit the needs of others and to claim Love. Even when other people try to point out to us that we are acting in ways that are not good for us, we are apt to drop the friends rather than confront our responses and the losses they hide. Responses that grow from our loss rather than our self-worth are so ingrained in us that we are unable to separate one from the other. I call these unhealthy and loss-induced emotional responses "guardian emotions." These emotions include the need to manipulate and control through blaming, resisting, bullying, judging, guilting, closing out, and siding with power.

## Guardian Emotions Cover Up
## Your Losses and Self-Worth

The term "guardian emotion" suggests a dichotomy. We think of a guardian as a helper, such as a guardian angel. We assume that the emotions we feel are accurate reflections of our circumstances. We've become comfortable with these old responses because they're familiar. They've been successful in the past in helping us rationalize our emotional pain and loss as we grew up. Guardian emotions, however, gain a momentum of their own, and we soon fail to realize the warp that has been built into our systems.

Guardian-emotion responses hide our self-worth and obstruct our inner vision. When we come up against old painful memories, all we feel are our guardian emotions, and these keep us away from our pain. Since our self-worth lies buried in our painful old memories, we consciously protect ourselves from finding what we most need: the truth.

When the bottom falls out of our lives in spiritual crisis and we are thrown into internal and often external turmoil, we are forced to challenge our assumptions about every part of our belief system. We are required to learn to respond from an honest inner world if we hope to evoke new levels of wellness.

We can authenticate our self-worth and develop a peaceful mind only when we learn the art of questioning our responses. When we learn to identify these old patterns, we're often amazed at their pervasiveness in all our relationships. We become free and able to bond with others without fear, jealousy, or anxiety as we search out and dismantle our destructive guardian emotions. This is a significant aspect to living in an emotionally responsible and healthy fashion.

As we each heal the pain from our emotional losses we become an asset rather than a liability to those around us. In releasing our guardian emotions we become true participants in life, building positive energy in our families and with all the people we chance to meet. This singular effort to release ourselves from self-destructive old emotions, when multiplied by many millions of people, translates into healing our planetary community.

## Why You Are in Spiritual Crisis

When we are in spiritual crisis, we are ready to change. We want to heal, so we need to identify what we truly feel, to know we are safe and secure in saying what we mean regardless of the responses of others, to set genuine personal boundaries so that our needs can be recognized. In this endeavor we unleash our self-worth, expanding our life-force energy toward healing and service.

One of the most immediate and pressing needs in healing is believing in ourselves and trusting our decisions. If we live with a person or people who are unlikely to accept our change or who insist on their view of truth and right action, then we'll have extra incentive to find others who share our desire for personal growth. We women have a particularly difficult time believing in the choices we make to facilitate our own change. We often have little experience in making the important decisions for our lives, so we're easily overwhelmed with the details of possible choices for our healing or recovery. But we are the ones who live with the benefit and consequences of our choices, and thus we learn that we can trust ourselves. It feels good to choose our directions, even if it is scary, and even if we decide later that we're ready to do the exact opposite.

As we begin to heal and honor our inner worth, we find that others are not really to blame for our struggles: we are the ones learning from our past and the present. The intimate and loving relationships we want to surround us are formed with those who are also working toward wholeness. We do have choices every day, and we make the right ones for our lives by believing in ourselves and accepting that we are meant to heal into joy and health. But as long as we stick with our guardian emotions, we attract those who also lead with theirs.

Is there a process we can engage in to begin untying our guardian emotion responses from our lives? Yes, but because our guardian emotions have become virtually undetectable, we'll need to pay close attention to our conversations and to give others we love and trust permission to help us change. We begin to change as we "catch" ourselves responding from the protection of our guardian emotions. When those emotions have taken over our responses, it is difficult to step aside, because we're caught in the energy of illusion. Yet with our new awareness we know more quickly when someone close to us has retreated into an angry, berating, whining, or victim-inspired dialogue. We can help ourselves, our family and friends, or others by agreeing to interrupt either our own dysfunctional patterns or those of others whenever they emerge.

Sometimes we think other people have it in for us when the culprit is really only our own paranoia. Other times, people may in fact have their own hidden agendas. While we can't control the responses others choose, we can choose the ways in which we perceive and respond in our lives to the actions of others. If a relationship has turned sour, if we're in the middle of a conversation and suddenly find ourselves covering our solar plexus and feeling uncomfortable, something has happened. We need to know what has transpired and why we've reacted as we have.

## The "Courage-to-Change" Bean Alert

In order to create a healthy body and the inner resources necessary to change and heal, we need to build energy from our acknowledged self-worth. I devised what I call the "Courage-to-Change" Bean Alert because I wanted a loving but effective method to help myself and others acknowledge old patterns that were getting in the way of productive, caring, and meaningful communication.

The purpose of this instant feedback system of giving someone black beans and hugs is to interrupt dysfunctional emotional patterns as they occur. Nothing is gained by prolonged arguing, getting angry at yourself, or trying to reason with a person who is responding from a stance protected by his or her guardian emotions. What is required is a quick and clear way to alert an individual that the conversation isn't helpful, enjoyable, or constructive. Literally handing that person a dried bean means "time out!" or "take a few breaths" or "let's talk in a different way."

When you try this exercise you'll know why I labeled it the "Courage-to-Change" Bean Alert. For most of us it takes great courage to openly acknowledge a destructive pattern of interaction with others and to ask for their help. It is equally difficult to give a bean to someone else, thereby acknowledging the presence of the person's destructive patterns. Yet taking this step to acknowledgment of the truth and requesting help can launch us toward meaningful change.

To initiate the "Courage-to-Change" Bean Alert, you as the person committed to sincerely wanting to see your own guardian emotions expelled, or you as the individual wanting to help a friend or colleague expel them, might begin by giving each person who will be participating in the process a handful of ordinary black cooking beans. Instruct people to keep them in a place from which they can be quickly retrieved, such as in a pocket, purse, or desk drawer. Advise them to give you a bean whenever they feel you are reverting to a pattern of conversation that is not leading to meaningful dialogue and is hurting your relationship.

When people can find ways to alert others to their distress, then communication can be expanded, new initiatives can be born, and the end result is that the individual or group becomes more respectful and responsive. This process also offers a way for people in partnerships to call attention to repressed feelings that most people, women especially, just try to live with. Many women feel that their partners are overbearing, controlling, and unwilling to listen or meet their needs. Men, too often, feel that their partners are unresponsive to their needs and push or nag them in ways that are counterproductive. And frequently we ostracize a person we find hard to work with or maneuver around someone we find difficult to be with.

We've all had the experience of leaving a job or even support or study group in which everyone is aware that one or two people are creating a problem for everyone else but no one wants to risk losing friendships or hurting feelings. The "Courage-to-Change" Bean Alert can help as part of a process for personal growth. Giving a bean allows you to disengage from a counterproductive conversation and take back your power while beginning a different, more meaningful conversation.

Expect that receiving a black bean from a partner, friend, or colleague feels like a face full of cold water. If you receive a bean, your response will either encourage the change process or squash it. Getting a bean doesn't mean that either you or the other person is wrong. It does mean the emotional atmosphere is not conducive to productive dialogue.

## Four Situations Calling for Change

I've identified four types of conversations in which giving a bean is helpful. Add your own experiences as you use this process or one of your own. Giving a bean is helpful:

1. when the exchange is heated and prolonged distress is apparent.

2. when the exchange is controlled, one-sided, and
   non-participatory.
3. when the exchange calls for positive assertion and
   leadership, but none is forthcoming.
4. when the exchange is stalled in argument.

When a bean is either given or received, the opportunity is there to stop the conversation and for each person to consider the ways in which he or she has contributed. We don't learn until we are ready and willing to make the effort and accept responsibility for our thoughts and actions. We change most easily when:

- we discover that others will not support the use of our old patterns.
- we want the love, respect, and positive feedback from others and realize that to get it, we must change.
- we can identify the difference between exchanges initiated from our goodness (self-worth) and those from our losses and inner pain.
- we understand that we are not our patterns, and that our goodness is present and available to us.
- we have some experience in living and sharing from our own goodness.
- we are encouraged by participation with others committed to both their own positive change and to facilitating our own.

## You Are Not Your Patterns

When we receive a bean, we are given notice by someone who cares about us that our guardian emotion patterns have replaced our self-worth as the basis for the emotional exchange. This means that what is running the conversation is our fearful emotional patterns rather than positive emotions stemming from our wisdom, compassion, openness, responsiveness, or self-love. Our job is to stop the old dysfunctional pattern in its cycle and make room for our goodness and self-worth to make itself known to us. Remember, we are not our patterns.

We all have experiences with others when their patterns are "on top" and when the real persons are no longer present. By giving a bean we ask a person to disengage from a pattern in order to give us his or her best, because we want and need that person and the person's perspective in our life and work.

I've often heard women claim that the men who emotionally berated or devalued them had a "different side," one below the surface of the behavior being displayed. The task for each of us is to accept that this "different side" is to be nurtured, because it is what makes us lovable and successful in our relationships and our lives.

The Courage-to-Change instant alert process for interrupting our patterns is extremely effective and at the same time emotionally strenuous. Being "caught in the act of using our patterns" may make us upset and angry. We will want to dismiss the process, blame others, get even, or just leave the group or gathering. Getting a bean feels rather like having the proverbial rug pulled out from under you.

The point of this exercise is, of course, to help each of us interrupt our patterns so that our own goodness is present more often than our defensive patterns. And when our guardian emotions do jump up, we can more easily acknowledge why we are responding the way we are.

# A Penetrating Look at Specific Guardian Emotions

When we give or receive a bean, it may mean that we are using one or more of the following guardian emotions to control or manipulate others:

## 1. Blaming

We blame people when we are afraid that we are inadequate. To point the finger at someone else takes the pressure off us. When we can keep the focus on the ways in which others caused the problem, or made a mistake, or did or said something that was the "real" difficulty, then we slide away from accepting responsibility and "ownership" in our part of the exchange.

The person who always blames others sees himself or herself as the victim, the one always getting the worst part of every deal. People who blame expect that their genuine efforts will ultimately be swept away unnoticed. They imagine and often create situations in which they are left unacknowledged, hurt, or undervalued. They expect life will always let them down, and so they set up the situations in which they give their power to others—and then resent it when others take it.

> *"It was Mary's idea to do it that way."*
>
> *"It's your fault we had that accident; I told you not to go out last night."*
>
> *"The raises were announced last night and, of course, I didn't get one. They never see the work I do."*
>
> *"There isn't a God, or life wouldn't be so painful."*

## 2. Resisting

We resist learning from or listening to others when we fear that they are always going to be right and we are always going to be wrong. We feel that others will always criticize us and that our attempts will always be considered inadequate. We usually create scenarios in which we appear to be the losers, the ones who must always capitulate to get ahead. In fact, we've often grown up in families in which a parent has been a domineering force, and in order to keep the Love we've needed, we've had to give in, although we felt we were right or justified in our actions. As adults we become obstinate in our resistance to others' suggestions because we've internalized this self-criticism.

> *"Why are you asking me about that job again? I've already done my best."*
>
> *"I'm not interested in excuses, I just want the job done right."*
>
> *"I don't want to hear your opinions on the reason I lost my job—my boss just had it in for me."*

### 3. Bullying

The person who is a bully has learned that if he or she makes enough "noise and commotion," others will stop pressing for change. Additionally, the person who resorts to emotional or physical bullying has found this approach a successful means of asserting superiority over others. That person thinks bullying makes him or her feel respected by others. If we've been bullied ourselves all our lives, then we learn bullying as a means of asserting our own authority.

This guardian emotion, like all the others, grows from having an underdeveloped sense of self-worth and feeling that if people get too close they will find it out. This guardian emotion causes us to atrophy emotionally because bullying allows us to use overpowering emotions to cover up our lack of worth, and consequently we lose touch with our gentler and more subtle emotions. We become unable to acknowledge that we feel, and can express directly, a different set of emotions: Love, compassion, pain, and fear.

> *"I don't have time to try and explain this to you again; just do it right this time."*
>
> *"You don't know anything—why are you so dumb?"*
>
> *"You always take things too seriously; you're too thin-skinned."*

## 4. Judging

This emotional response is present in about 99.9 percent of adults. We accept that we have a right to run down and dissect the actions and character of others when they are not around. We do this when we need reassurance that we are better than others: smarter, better looking, more appealing, wiser, more practical, or whatever the criteria in question. When we are unsure of our value we need others to continually prop us up with reassurances. The best way for us to continually elicit other people's reassurances of our ability and their Love or respect for us is to put ourselves in a competition or comparison mode with others. Often, people who judge others have felt judged in their growing-up years—and they believed they never measured up to the expectation others held.

> *"I can't do my job because Joyce has a bad attitude and is impossible to work with."*
>
> *"Pam was so hard to get along with last night—I wouldn't talk to someone that way."*
>
> *"Peter is so insecure and self-centered."*

## 5. Guilting

When people use guilt on us as a means of getting their

needs met, we know we don't feel good about the conversation but may not understand why. The person who uses guilt knows that by re-stimulating certain inner chords of fear, pain, lack of Love, or anxiety, that person can get his or her way. Parents are often accused by their children of using this guardian emotion. Guilt is an especially difficult emotion to expose because it is camouflaged within genuine feelings and is just about impossible for us to counter effectively.

If anxieties are expressed by innuendo or suggestion rather than directly, you can assume the person is afraid to tell you outright what he or she needs and so must cloak those needs in a way that permits them to be slid into the conversation and into your mind. People who use guilt do so because they've never been allowed to acknowledge their own needs.

> *"I have so much work to do that I have to work longer than anyone else."*

> *"If you loved me you would come for dinner."*

> *"It's too bad that you're so busy that you don't have time for your family."*

### 6. Closing Out

This guardian emotion uses rhetorical questions to coerce others into agreement or at least silence. People who use this closing-out technique do so from a fear of conflict. Many people who seem well-adjusted and self-contained use this guardian emotion effectively. They get people to go along with their ideas because they seem so positive and forthright that any disagreement would seem unacceptable.

Often, people who use closing out as part of their conversation talk quickly and animatedly, moving from one subject to the next without pauses or room for discussion. People use this when their experience has taught them that disagreement leads quickly and inevitably to serious conflict and perhaps even emotional or physical violence.

> *"Everything is going so wonderfully, I'm sure you must feel terrific about our progress."*
>
> *"Don't you just love this new idea?"*
>
> *"I'm sure we can raise the necessary money, and here is my plan."*

## 7. Denying

People who use this guardian emotion feel safer in the world of illusion, where all things are only mutable forces. When we use denial we are saying that we are comfortable being a shadow, not responsible for our words or actions and out of touch with reality. We deny our motives or actions when we are afraid to assert an opinion or to feel justified in thinking at all. We deny our real intentions in order not to make a target for others.

The guardian emotion of denying usually comes from growing up in an atmosphere in which our thoughts, intentions, or actions were misunderstood or devalued. We decided somewhere deep inside that it was safer never to give people a chance to belittle us, and so we became the shadow.

> *"I didn't say he couldn't go, just that he probably wouldn't want to."*
>
> *"I'm sure this pain isn't anything and will go away."*
>
> *"It doesn't matter to me whether you do or don't take the job."*

**8.  *Siding with Power***

This guardian emotion allows us to always be right because in every argument or discussion we side with those who we think hold the power.  Our response comes from lining up with those who we think will win so that we will win by association.  Children often do this in families where there is physical abuse and where children choose the side of the parent who seems to carry the power.  With this guardian emotion in control, we never put ourselves out of alignment with the assumed power force either at work or at home.

This guardian emotion response is often reinforced through experiences in which we did try to stand up to a person or "the system" and were laughed at, humiliated in some way, or hurt physically.  Memories like these are etched in our minds forever.  We decide it's safe only to agree with the opinion and actions of those in power.  We don't want to be different, because to stand out is dangerous.

*"You and I understand how things are around here."*

*"It doesn't matter what they say, I'll back you up."*

*"I'm sure you're right, that person's no good."*


## Challenging Your Old Patterns

While I've mentioned only some of the more obvious guardian emotions, you'll come to identify many more.  Guardian emotions come in clusters, so many of the ones I've described may seem relevant to you.  Not all guardian emotions are acted out in loud, angry, or dismissive tones.  Some of the most destructive ones are pressed on us with a smile or a quiet tone of voice.  We all have different means through which we manipulate and control others to get our needs met.  We've developed these responses in an effort to sidestep our reality and create the caring, loving, and supportive environment we need.

Some people's patterns are especially difficult for us to be around. This often means that in the past these same patterns were used on us, or that we've had direct and unpleasant association with them. Yet when we break through guardian emotions that tie us to certain behavior, we find we are also untied from those who use them. Others can be our "teachers" when they call to our attention places where we are still attached to certain guardian emotions. When we are joined to others by our guardian emotions, we are held as tightly as two pieces of velcro. When we remove our own connection to a pattern, we cut away the velcro. Because it takes two pieces of velcro to make a connection, when you heal your half of the conflict by healing your guardian emotion you are freed so that the situation has the room to change.

If a conversation isn't mutually informative or helpful, then both people have a responsibility to discover why. When we are calmly in control of our responses, all of this seems reasonable, but when we are upset or feeling totally justified in our response, we may find it difficult to have someone suggest that we are not expressing ourselves out of our own inner worth but out of our fear and pain. It takes courage to give a bean, and it takes courage to accept one.

If we can remember that our patterns are the deflected emotional responses we've always used to keep people away from our emotional losses and fears, then we can see how getting a bean can be an upsetting experience. We've used these deflective emotional responses in the past to meet our needs and to cover up our inadequacies. When a pattern is interrupted, like a live electric wire waving in the breeze it needs to be re-connected to a desirable new line in order for the energy to begin to flow in a more productive direction.

Give hugs as well as beans! Be sure to show people that you see their progress and their efforts by giving hugs as well as beans. Part of the change process of growing emotionally and spiritually involves calling someone's attention to those actions that are destructive. The balancing part in this formula for change is to also offer a steady stream of praise, hugs, and affirmations of the positive changes in individuals' attitudes and behavior.

Change becomes possible through simple programs like this Courage-to-Change Bean Alert. We can identify and encourage healing in ourselves and others in ways that honor us both as well as the process of becoming whole. We have choices, and these include either allowing our relationships to wallow in guardian emotions or challenging our old patterns in order to find and live from our self-worth. Your healing depends on shifting to the latter.

# 10 Building a Personal Relationship with the God-force

*Whenever you surrender, you give in not
to the pain in your life but to the force
that pushes you through the pain or
the pain through you.*

We heal only when we accept that we are part of a larger force. Healing is an expansion of ourselves into a different kind of Love and self-acceptance. As we learn to awaken these powerful feelings, we attract complementary energy from the God-force, the Universal system. In order to heal we need an unshakeable belief in our place within a greater field of loving energy. This awareness, when acted upon, furthers the usable energy in our own life systems for healing and recovery and also helps us fill in the losses and fears that cause us to be "energy sieves."

Spiritual energy comes from our use of spiritual tools, those that remind us of God and the ways to use the universal principles that support all life. Where have we come from, and where will we go when we leave this life? We don't usually stop to consider these questions until we must, or until we are deciding whether or not we want the life that we have. We each experienced being born, though we don't consciously remember it, and we'll all experience dying. We are deeply moved by the miracle of life when we watch a child born, when we see life when it is new and untarnished, not weighted down by life's struggles, and feel that something of great beauty and value has come from beyond physical form. When we stand beside the grave of someone we've loved, we experience in reverse the same sensation we've acknowledged at birth: something beautiful and of great value has again moved beyond physical form. We are left to ponder the meaning of it all.

Any religious tradition can lead us to the all-encompassing living environment that encourages the focusing of our attention on God. Many of us left a church or temple, or left it with our hearts, when we felt traditional doctrine was insufficient to address our spiritual needs or those of humanity. Many of us felt we didn't receive the spiritual guidance for which we hungered. We were told to believe or else, and this felt too much like man-made rules.

When we are in spiritual crisis we're looking to find or re-create a relationship with the God-force that is built on more than systems of dogma or punitive responses to humankind's supposed "sins." Surely, there is a God-force that loves all equally, and alignment with this expansive source of Love can help us heal our hearts and mend our broken planet.

## Weeding Out Beliefs that Hold No Power

When in spiritual crisis we want to find conviction and trust but may be unsure where to begin. We do know that our current view of creation and the forces of the Universe are too distant to give us comfort. We want a personal relationship, and we want it to be based on truth and acceptance of our struggle. As we search for the ropes to hold us, to weave together a trusted bed of grace for our recovery, we must untangle and remove the beliefs that are false to us, that hold no power. We can only build on the truth that we hold in our hearts, and all that we read and learn must resonate with what "feels true for us."

## Seeing God as the Parent and Trying to Bargain

We develop and reinforce our beliefs about the Universe according to the success and failure we've had when trying to heal, help, or in some way control our lives. When we pray for a loved one to be returned to us from a coma, or walk the floor an hour after a teenager's curfew asking that he or she be returned to us safely, or mumble a few silent promises when we open the envelope and read the letter that tells us whether or not we passed or succeeded in certain ways, we are bargaining with Divine Providence to do things our way.

As we see our prayers answered or not, we settle on a working understanding of the Universe. We offer assurances that we are worthy of this thing we are asking for, that we will take care of this person, make good in this job, never do another ugly thing, if just this once we can be saved or helped. These are promises just like the ones we felt obliged to make to our parents when we were growing up. If life registers in the "comfort zone," then we think God is smiling on us.  If it registers in the "misery zone," then we think God has forgotten us.  Seeing God in this way is seeing the Divinity of our childhood; this is God as the parent.

We try to anticipate God's responses to our prayers and seek to do the things that we think will make a difference so that we can stay in control.  But thinking isn't linked to the energy of the Universe; inner knowing is.  And fear of losing control of our lives is only a mental construct.  It is like the fear of falling backward into the waiting arms of a friend.  What if the friend  moves, what if we get dropped, what if we're hurt—but what if we're caught?

Many people have a nagging inner voice inherited from their religious upbringing that makes transitioning out of fear, guilt, and unworthiness extremely difficult.  We may for many years go through the motions of changing our inner landscape while still preserving our search at the mental level.  But when we are in disease or severe loss, our search through old beliefs to a fresh, meaningful perspective becomes a necessity for physical survival.  No quick and easy method will do in our spiritual journey.  Our lives may have come down to this point:  what do we believe, and of what use is it to us in this life?

It is easy to continue to see God as the parent because such a view gives us someone to blame when things don't work out, and we have a source from which the miraculous can still rescue us.  To take on a belief in God on our own terms as a partner more than a parent is scary and seemingly presumptuous.

## Feeling You Have No Right to Direct Experience of God's Love

Many religions teach us to feel unworthy in our relationships with the Divine.  Feeling unworthy means we have no right to know God. The way to develop spiritual independence is the good old trial-and-error method. The only way to build personal spiritual power is to try on different ideas for size, work them through, sit with them, and come to know your relationship with the Sacred. One of the most difficult challenges we face in life is trying to sort out what we believe about God. Yet if we are to move out of spiritual crisis, rebuilding our lives in a more stable and meaningful way, then defining our feelings about the Divine is critical.

A client named Melinda experienced the God-force at work in her life when she became pregnant with the child she was afraid to have. She was ambivalent about having this child because she felt so unsteady in her own life. She felt too confused to consider the added responsibility of a child. But in spite of the herbs she had taken during the first two months of her pregnancy to initiate a miscarriage, the fetus stayed in her uterus. By the time she was three months pregnant, she had a change of heart, literally, and decided she really wanted the child simply because she felt its presence inside her and knew that something unexplainable and miraculous was happening.

When we uncork our fears and expectations of God and allow God to speak to us in the middle of confusion, we find a clearer path toward meaningful solutions for our lives. Often, we feel the presence of the God-force in a joyful moment, a beautiful experience, a powerful instant of inner certainty that needs no further definition, only acknowledgment that this may be the God-force at work in our lives.

## Assuming the God-force Responds in Human Ways

Maturing into a new phase of spirituality begins with accepting that events are not within our control, nor should they be. After all, should we assume that all the laws of creation should change according to our desired outcome? To want this is to want a God-force and Universal principles that can be manipulated, for good reasons or bad. Part of our struggle comes from believing that if the Universe is based on Love, then we can see no reason for not getting what we are praying for: what harm would it do? We deserve it, we've tried or worked hard for this thing. Or the person who is dying doesn't deserve to die.

When we pray for help and feel we've done our part and then have been let down, we want to know who has the answers and who is to blame. It is extremely difficult to avoid the natural response of assuming that the God-force responds in human ways. When we do our part and keep doing our part, then it means we're committed to learning, not just correcting one situation. A client of mine who had periodic panic attacks sought spiritual guidance initially as a means of putting out these firey episodes. Through our working together she began to develop a support network that helped her learn to work with spiritual energy on a continuing basis. She began to feel calmer and less prone to the peaks and valleys of instant fear and instant freedom from fear.

## Taking the Leap of Faith

When we have painful or even life-threatening experiences, we want to know why. We have a choice of whom to blame: either God or ourselves. And when it is too scary to blame God, we blame ourselves or others. These questions of ultimate responsibility are not easily answered and are probably not meant to be. If we do have the courage to blame God, if we are willing to risk that the totality of our beliefs may burn up in the fury of our anger at the injustice of our situation or the overwhelming pain of our loss, then maybe we can "hear" the voice of truth from the Universe. Because in acknowledging that, in fact, we do blame God for letting this misery befall us, we are honest in our pain, and we are asking to be shown the true presence of Divinity. We have been willing to empty out the old opinions and to have nothing, trusting that this openness and emptiness will lead to something different and better.

To answer any question that involves the Divine Source requires a passage into a different inner space, where answers are gifts and questions are the bearer of those gifts. In other words, we cannot possibly expect that God is going to produce answers on demand, but we can stretch our expectations for instant resolution in order for insight to come to us in the way of the Universe: all in good time. In this more accepting frame of mind we gradually come to value the Divine presence as more than the giver of joy, health, and satisfaction or the taker away of these same human needs. We find that the God-force is the source of the eternal questions in our lives, requiring us to stretch and change our beliefs to find relationship with a continually changing Universe.

## Shifting to a Love-Based Relationship

The teachings of many religious traditions assert that if their teachers control a child until the age of seven, the child will forever after be a believer. We are impressionable when young and often come to believe that God, like our parents, operates according to a reward-and-punishment system. When we are good, God will love us, and when we are bad, God will punish us. But what does that mean? What does it mean to be good or bad? Who is setting the standards: our parents? God?

As children we are taught our parents' ideology—
except that we are told it is the absolute truth. And if we
are to be saved, or if we are good boys or girls, we too will
accept this belief package without question. To question
this package is in some religions tantamount to heresy. To
accept without reservation or resistance is held up as the
ideal for which all should strive. Because God figures so
significantly in most people's lives, the disasters that befall
us are quickly seen as obvious punishments for some
known or unknown transgression.

As adults, however, we are required to free ourselves
from the imprinting that tells us that our relationship with
the Divine is built on fear rather than Love. Fear lies inside
many hearts: fear of doing the wrong thing, fear that we
are undeserving of Love unless we do certain things for
others, fear that we are not good enough or inherently
important enough to call on the God-force.

Children figure that because God is so important, punishment for failing to be a true believer will be imposed in
devastating ways. A death in the family, divorce, failure in
school, or lack of peer support stay imbedded in a young
person's consciousness as punishment deserved from a Universe he or she has come to fear.

Children need to have the chance to grow in a healthy
way by being encouraged to see God as a source of Love
that doesn't punish, that hurts when we hurt, that forgives,
and that continually teaches us of the highest values and
goals that sustain all manner of life. This is the belief system in which there are no human-made absolutes but
where we and God are in partnership. We possess sparks
or droplets of Divinity equally as pure as those of the God-
force because they are extensions of the God-force. These
droplets are our souls, and our souls continually put forth

the energy that can change and heal our lives.

We are manipulated easier and controlled easier with fear than we can be with Love. Love is open-ended, given without reservation. Fear is the opposite, and we cannot give Love if we are afraid of being loved or feel undeserving of Love. Because we are taught through some religions or by some of our elders that the Creator capriciously gives or withholds Love, we come to give and trust Love in our personal relationships as a reflection of these beliefs.

Children come into this world in small human forms, but they have full-sized souls. If our belief in a God-force is fear-based rather than acceptance- and love-based, then we set up an internal duality of belief that will affect our lives until we change our views. Because we come into this world from the world of spirit, the world of oneness and alignment with the Almighty, we are not evil or tarnished but pure loving beings intent upon earthly experiences and learnings. This means that if we are taught a doctrine based on fear, that doctrine is in direct opposition to what our childhood souls know intuitively to be true. Because the child's soul is fully capable of holding Love, it is searching for the ways to gather Love while it is part of a physical body in this earthly existence. All children know this whether raised as Buddhists, Jews, Muslims, Christians, or as a member of some other religious tradition.

Your journey through spiritual crisis and the dark night of the soul is bent on reuniting you with the parts of your inner self that have become separated from you as you strove to meet your parents' expectations or to adopt beliefs that taught you only a fear-based doctrine. The God-force is Love. Your soul's challenge is to grow in Love by finding self-love and allowing the Universe to match this with its own force for healing.

## Re-Examining Guilt as Your Prime Motivator

Who hasn't felt guilty about doing something or failing to do something that in our heart of hearts we knew was wrong? Through intention or action we perhaps did something questionable to our children, or failed to handle a sticky situation in a good way, or betrayed someone we loved. Maybe we hurt another person or many people in a way that haunts our nights and tears at our inner sense of self.

Prolonged guilt is one of our most destructive human responses because it's futile. Like locking the proverbial barn door after the horse has been stolen, we respond in the months and even years after the fact, reliving and replaying those feelings that we sidestepped, ignored, or buried when we made certain critical choices. We may feel that we can never again truly reclaim our honorable or empowered personhood.

Guilt plays a big part in our learning to trust God, in our willingness to again trust ourselves, and in our challenge of claiming a spiritual perspective that both holds us accountable and also offers forgiveness.

Religion has for centuries coerced people into accepting that they were separate from God and that those who spoke for the church were the only ones who could forgive in the name of God. Many have been taught to believe that God requires punishment for wrongdoing and that some crimes are never forgivable. Do these thoughts make sense to us today? Do they still feel right as we turn them around inside? Are we forever held to a Universe that causes us misery and withholds the soothing hand of forgiveness? I think not.

What would it mean to be truly separate from the Universe? We would die, because like a baby born without a heart, we could not fulfill our work here on Earth. If we were separate from the God-force we would need to figure out ways to regain our connection. If we were separate we might need others to tell us the ways to again become reunited with this benevolent force. But we are not separate. We are simply unaware that this bond is present. We don't need to create it; we need only recognize and use it.

We have lived too long expecting others to make our choices, to fix our lives, to tell us what to believe and how to be forgiven. And we have gone far too deeply into the creation of our culture without realizing that we require no spiritual intercession; we and the Universe are one, forever united and aligned.

When we think and act in ways that go contrary to the laws of the Universe, we feel the direct hit of the Universe's energy through our hearts. This is what we interpret as guilt: "I could have, should have" thoughts. The "if only" responses are those that hold us in guilt. When we do something that goes against our God-space, we hurt, and that is a good thing. When we hurt, it means that we have failed in some way to value another or many others and have not upheld our responsibility to participate in life-supporting action to the best of our ability. We do hurt ourselves when we hurt another because we have intentionally or inadvertently trampled on another's heart.

## Learning to Live in Right Relationship with the Divine

Trusting the God-force comes from success in making choices for our lives that feel fulfilling. A two-year-old is prepared to decide whether he or she wants a cookie with or without a cup of juice, not whether he or she will be a painter, teacher, or salesperson when grown up. Trusting the Universe also comes from feeling prepared for those big choices that we face. In spiritual crisis we feel ill-prepared for the upsetting, maybe even devastating, circumstances we find ourselves in. The situation in our physical lives only mirrors the ambivalence and disillusionment we may feel with God.

Spiritual preparedness grows from genuine personal experience with Divinity. Guilt can either hold us in a morass of destructive feelings or can propel us toward our real challenge that speaks to the issue of free choice and essential spiritual preparation for life choices.

As children we may not have been given choice as to our spiritual education. When we're young we're sent to school to learn the basics before we are expected to go on to high school, college, or graduate school. When we begin to learn about the Universe through a spiritual tradition, we may also attend religious training. Does this training help us develop our own model for living in right relationship with the Divine? Does this spiritual work give us the push to ask our own questions, to find God in our own way? Usually, the answer is "no." We are given a cursory understanding only of what our religion and those in authority expect from us, and through this voice we are to interpret the true nature of God. We live with this second-hand view of God until we face deep enough guilt, severe enough anguish, that we bottom out, breaking through our complacency, confronting our spiritual uncertainty.

Life is a cumulative experience; we confront, we're in pain, we learn, we grow, we build anew. We are foolish if we expect our lives to miss one of these essential beats. Wisdom comes, rather, from watching the cycle at work in our lives and from partaking in a more meaningful way of the blessings we already possess. We don't earn life here on the Earth; we are given it. Likewise, we each have a different life path to play out, and the choices we make daily cause us to gain or lose energy and spiritually expand or contract according to the choices we make. Those embarking on the path of personal growth are best advised to watch this amazing process of change unfold within their lives and to honor it, knowing they cannot control it.

## Stepping through Anger to Transform Your Heart

Anger is often a response to guilt. Rather than feeling responsible for the outcome, the angry person feels the victim of life's experiences. We've all found ourselves overwhelmed at one point or another with anger, maybe even rage. Is anger a positive response or a negative one? Does it help or hurt us?

Anger can be a good thing, a means of cleansing ourselves of poisonous feelings. But prolonged anger coming from unresolved feelings corrodes our capacity to love and trust, inevitably leading us away from a positive re-entry into life.

When we accept that we are angry we are taking responsibility for rewriting the rules by which we will live. When we honor our anger and then work to release it, we let go of the risk of forever defining ourselves in terms of that anger. Anger focuses our attention on the underbelly of our lives, the places where we feel hurt, lacking, unworthy, less than we were intended to be. Eventually, we can become that anger and that pain. We can live so long with feelings that God deserted us, that life overwhelmed us, that we didn't deserve the outcome, that we can never again be happy, that we convince ourselves of the truth of our continued pain.

When we are hurting from a dramatic change in our lives, it is hard to see that the change is representative of something much bigger on our spiritual journey. When we feel like victims we can ask ourselves: Who made the rules by which we are playing and by which we've become the victim? Were the rules handed down to us, or did we help create them? Did we believe that others would look out for us or that our lives would magically just take care of themselves? Did we think that God would take care of us and that therefore pain and misery would never darken our doors? Did we think that loving others was a replacement for loving ourselves? Did our own needs go unanswered for too long, and do we believe that we are now meant to fulfill them ourselves?

Yes, the Universe pushes us to our limits. Sometimes we feel dangerously close to a place past our limits. But when we begin to build our spiritual edifice to withstand the hurricane-force winds of life, and we anchor our trust in the Universe rather than in life or other people, we will never again be confounded. Although our lives are dashed in many ways, when we have experience with an inner Divine force in our lives we can withstand anything and still survive and prosper.

Anger helps us clean up past miseries so that we can find God. Anger releases old poisons and pains so that we can be fresh and new, capable of again experiencing life with added perspective. We can use anger productively to rid ourselves of what no longer holds value in our lives. The Universe calls to each of us to know its presence and force in ways we are never initially prepared to understand or handle. We are apprenticed to the Creator, and the learnings to which we aspire are held out to us. Our choice is in the way we will accept these offerings: as pain or as joy, as death or as life, as loss or as transformation.

Anger has many sides: the need for self-love, hunger for appreciation, resentment for having life be unfair. Our feelings of anger can push deep into the soil of our lives and, with the Universe's help, transform our hurts into life-enhancing feelings that will grow new greenery.

We are learning to be avatars, teachers inspired by the wisdom of the Infinite, in order to help and heal our lives and the lives of many others. Our feelings lead us more deeply toward the inner facets of our soul.

## Understanding and Amplifying the Energy of Your Spirit

Each of us has a body, a mind, and a soul. All three aspects must work together if we are to be healthy, at peace, and able to learn from our experiences. Spirit is the energy of Love that fills our souls. Spirit, the Divine presence, is with us throughout our lives. We tend to think of spirit as amorphous, unreal, and only a religious or spiritual symbol. Yet spirit can attest to our purposes in this life, to our history as an immortal presence, and to a future that we are creating daily.

We cannot destroy our spirits by means of deceitful thoughts or actions. But we can amplify the force and effectiveness of this subtle energy through our use of Love, compassion, and right action. When we increase the amount of spiritual energy in our bodies, we can call on it for use by ourselves as well as to help and heal others. The energy of spirit is Love.

We feel the energy of our spirits at various times in our lives. We experience it as joy, as inner peace and well-being, as resolve and acceptance of change and loss. We also recognize the energy of spirit as that part of us that knows when a stage of our lives is over, even though we don't want it to be. When we feel sad and lonely, sick, unable to cope with the burdens of life, or confused about our future, or about the lack of guidance or direction or relationship with God, it means that we are not benefitting from the Love our spirits can inspire. Our minds are the arbitrators, the reflectors, the compilers, and the implementors. Our spirits are the creators. Only our spirits link us with the vast resources of the Universe; our minds, as part of the earthly living experience, simply stay with our bodies.

Our responsibility is to learn as much as we can about our lives, our thinking and feeling, and most of all our perception of the vast creativity that lies just under the surface of our conscious attention. If we are to contribute to the potpourri of positive growth and development on the Earth, then we must do our own homework to learn the tools of tomorrow's world that will be based on intuition, perception, and the unleashing of creativity that benefits all life.

When I work with people on their own healing, I find myself relating to soul and spiritual energy over and over again, because I believe deeply that it is in activating this link to the Divine that we can draw on the magnificent power and enlightenment of God for every part of our lives and for the life of the planet and all her creatures.

## Living the Spiritual Way

Nothing rational in your life is going to tell you how to awaken the spiritual in your life. You will need to accept that you are being shown your spiritual path right now; you are being given opportunities to further your understanding of God at this very moment, and once you begin, the next and then the next levels of understanding will become available to you.

Growing spiritually is a process rather than a goal. And the first step is to recognize that you are undergoing a spiritual change, a potentially life-transforming shift and readjustment. Realize that this is your wake-up call to a better understanding of the laws of the Universe first and to the needs and wants of humanity second.

You can begin to heal only when you realize that your life's crises contain your opportunity to become renewed, to be formed in a new way. This is the largest leap of faith that is required, because all the other changes essential for spiritual growth come in response to obvious challenges and to ordinary life situations that you can see and increasingly recognize as the Universe speaking to you in your daily life.

We find the God-force each in our own way, sometimes through powerful personal experiences and sometimes through a leap of faith that gives God no face but a presence in our lives that we trust. We find the God-force through our compassion for fellow human beings and other living things. As we reach out to trust life and to trust others, we feel less alone. As we gather with others to live in a sacred way, we encourage our spiritual search and discover a more profound and truer basis for our lives and our work. While we may begin our journey through spiritual crisis with little focus, we quickly discover the power that comes from sharing ideas, insights, and healing energy. We may have drawn people together in Love to help us, or we may be drawn to others to help; either way, we've responded to the central theme of life and Divinity—the capacity to love.

As we grow spiritually, we build the energy of our spirits automatically. The path that we prioritize becomes our path and source of energy. In paying attention to the consistently loving ways of the Universe, we are less fractured by the random ways of human beings.

Living in a spiritual way means accepting that we are part of the Universe, that all manner of life is interconnected.

We are bonded to other people and to our past and our future. We can recognize this and learn from this connection as we integrate these essential ingredients into our spiritual development:

- ability to love
- desire to share and learn with others
- willingness to be honest in our need of specific help or insight
- taking care of self and the Earth
- assuming responsibility for our actions and thoughts
- willingness to make the effort to separate dysfunctional attitudes from those perpetuated by feelings of self-worth
- ability to hear appropriately-stated critical evaluation
- willingness to yield the floor to others
- making an effort to live in spiritual optimism, one day at a time
- performing acts of selflessness and service.

Integrating these ways of being and living help us expand the positive flow of spiritual energy into our bodies, feelings, and thoughts, and also to hold on to the energy we have generated. At times of spiritual crisis, when we hope to learn the ways to correct our imbalances, we are wise to allow our spirits to lead the way toward a direct, personally meaningful relationship with the God-force.

# 11 Working with Energy to Heal the Physical Body

*Whenever you lovingly place your hands on another person, healing takes place on the most appropriate levels.*

The body-mind-spirit method of healing is based on ancient teachings that identified the healing power of this integrated approach. Popular holistic healing methods like Yoga, Tai Chi, Polarity, Rolfing, Regression, Massage, Iridology, Herbology, Naturopathy, Chiropractic or Osteopathic manipulation, Acupuncture, Kinesiology, Feldenkrais, Radionics, Color therapy, Crystal therapy, Mineral therapy, and Astrology all offer perspectives on healing. As I've stressed in this book, our total well-being depends on a healthy emotional interaction with others and our environment, an active spiritual exchange with the God-Force, and an engaged body wisdom that flushes imperfections from the system.

Some people respond more effectively to energy work

than others. The degree of positive response seems to be based partly on our belief in the power of either holistic or traditional models of health care. It may be a long reach for people to realize that simply taking drugs and medicines isn't enough to eliminate disease or long-standing distress from the body. An approach that identifies difficulty and healing opportunity in all three levels of ourselves will give us the most complete, long-lasting, and satisfactory results.

We are each responsible for giving and gaining all that we need from the methods of healing that we choose. Most health care  practitioners increasingly accept and encourage client involvement, as they should. I find it important to realize that when we go to a health practitioner, physician, nurse, therapist,  or body worker for any manner of work, either in a traditional vein or otherwise, we are helping each other. This means that we are giving the professional healer/health care practitioner an opportunity to be of service, using his or her specific skills. In turn, we benefit from the exchange of energy and insight from the skilled person. A mutual exchange of respect and Love is the ideal environment for healing, because as the patients we feel supported in seeking to assume responsibility for directing our own healing and for creating our own healing wheels.

## You'll Know If You Are Inclined to Work as a Healer

Every one of us has an innate desire to be of assistance to others. Sometimes this inner need is expressed in the desire to work with people at the "ideas" level; at other times we want to work with the physical body. When I talk about energy work in this book, I'm talking about working with a person's physical body to awaken all three levels of energy: body, mind, and spirit.

Since my earliest recollections I've had a sincere desire to work with people, beginning with volunteer work as a teenager in the children's ward of a nearby hospital. After college I seriously considered going to medical school. Then, when that didn't fall into place, years later I applied and was accepted for a graduate degree in nursing. Life complications and the adoption of our second child, a daughter, pushed this program out of reach. So I continued to hunger for ways to apply my intense desire to work in healing. In retrospect, I realize that the years of looking for my work weren't wasted. My various jobs all gave me a piece of my healing work, even though I didn't know that at the time. As so often happens, when we aren't looking to discover our lifework, we find it. My first book, *Agartha: A Journey to the Stars*,[1] chronicles my experiences with initiation into the world of spirituality and my awakening as an intuitive and healer.

## Healing Work Is Not Doing, It is Allowing

When we work with life-force energy, we invoke our intuitive knowing and our mental, emotional, and spiritual insight and wisdom to help an individual grow, change, and heal. I find that directing energy through our hands to another person is a meaningful and useful way to work. I've learned about energy and the nature of healing from my own spiritual work as well as from clients who have shared with me this spiritual journey toward wholeness.

As people change, their transformation is a cause for celebration. When they heal physically, it causes us feelings of enormous gratitude and awe for the process that is often possible. And when they die, it is a time of sadness for those of us left without them and also a time of quiet joy, because we can take comfort in knowing that they have moved beyond this place of time and space to a reality ever so much grander.

Healing has many dimensions. We need not be confined to any level of limitation for what we can expect,
because our bodies are meant to be healthy and whole and
our spirits are meant to participate in the fulfillment of that
objective. When I work with healing energy it is not
against the laws of the Universe or of Nature but with them.
The only reality that is being defied is that of self-limitation
and resistance to the obvious need to awaken access to the
greatest source and level of Love. As we do this we have
no need to control, direct, or force a person or situation to
capitulate; we merely allow the force and presence of the
Divine to flow through us to the person in need of it, to be
used by that person's own body wisdom for his or her best
and most appropriate use. This can mean we allow our
Love to merge with a greater Love in order to direct specific
attention to a person or specifically to a person's organs or
systems that are in pain and out of balance. It is not
through our doing, but through our allowing, that the Love
of the Universe pushes aside grief and distress and awakens
joy and inner balance.

## Etheric Energy and Body Wisdom

You may remember, etheric energy is the level of energy
connected most closely with the physical body. Etheric
energy contains the blueprint of perfect health for the body.
While we can't see etheric energy, we can sense it in others
by placing our hands close to their bodies. We can sense
our own etheric energy through a force or pulse I call the
body wisdom. This sound current, beat, or pulse unites the
organs, keeping them aware of their purpose and helping
them work in harmony for the total health of the body.
This sound presence filters through the physical body,

maintaining the appropriate healing balance. When this beat or pulse becomes diminished through trauma or disease, the essential energy flow among organs and systems of the body slows down, and eventually, if disease or trauma become severe enough, the resonance ceases, and the person dies.

People identify this sound, or body-wisdom pulse, in various ways. Some sense it as a familiar sound from their childhood, one that has positive connotations connected with people or experiences they've loved, like the sound of wind in the trees. Others sense it as a definite pulse or color wave, or as ripples in a small pond. Still others talk about feeling it as a silent but benevolent presence.

In seeking to restore balance to our bodies, we benefit when our healing coach works with our energy fields to heighten and help restore our body wisdom's pulse.

## Working with a Person's Body Wisdom

If you are interested in having your healing coach help restore your body wisdom, or if you feel the desire to work on someone you love, the following thoughts and instructions can be useful. For most people, it takes time and practice to "sense" another person's body wisdom, yet if you understand how to work with energy and understand what is happening, you can quickly become an effective healer.

The body wisdom pulse originates in the area of the solar plexus. Before working on a person, it's important to tune into the person's rhythm, general emotional state, and body language. By taking a few minutes to do this you are more apt to be successful when going on to work with organs in the ways most effective for alleviating specific pain and other distressing symptoms. After this initial attunement the healer is free to place his or her hands on the client's solar plexus, working in ever-expanding concentric circles from the mid-point of the solar plexus outward. Sometimes I place my left hand in the small of the person's back while I'm working with my right hand on his or her mid-section. This seems to give me even more of a sensitive feeling about the person's needs and the directions my hands should move.

This first initiative to awaken and get to know the client's body wisdom may also be enough to restore a normal level of energy exchange among the organs. Often, however, when moving to work with specific organs the healer discovers that the organs or systems that are under stress from disease or dysfunction are lacking the pulse emanating from the body wisdom. In this case, the healer must go back to the solar plexus and work in this area until sufficient energy has been generated to allow the distressed organ(s) to again pick up the beat. The length of time that it takes for an organ to respond gives the healer an indication of the extent of the disease. Twenty to forty-five minutes is usually sufficient to restore an organ to alignment with the body wisdom, even an organ that is seriously impaired from, for example, a cancer tumor.

## How Body Wisdom Is Influenced by Emotions and Healing Energy

A progressive disease may seem to be worse than it actually is because pain interrupts the body wisdom's bonding pulse and so literally cuts off the organ(s) from the rest of the system. This increases the organ's distress considerably. The person in distress feels increased lethargy, depression, pressure at the point of the tumor or disease, and a general decrease in overall well-being. This is because organs are able to move energy among themselves and to take on a greater load when one organ has trouble. When an organ is cut off from this support, it deteriorates quickly. If an organ still has the capacity to heal, it will be able to again pick up the body wisdom pulse, and the healer will feel the reflection of this energy back through his or her hands.

In working in this way you are drawing forth the person's innate body wisdom so that the organs have increased access to this energy after you've stopped working on them. A person's body wisdom is essential to the healing process and is the basic force that orchestrates and maintains equilibrium and the flow of healing energies among organs and systems. It also encourages the body's detection of disease so that when this happens, the disease is recognized as foreign and undesirable, and the body's immune responses can be called into action.

Many cancers, for instance, are not detected by the body as a destructive or life-threatening force. This means that one's body wisdom has accepted the intruder because it is aligned with emotions that the person accepts as part of his or her life. Negative and loss-oriented emotions of our past attract and hold in place the diseases in our current lives. If you are afraid, aren't sure of your future, feel unhappy or unloved or out of step with your life, then those emotions are translated to your body. A person's body wisdom can override short-term traumas and distresses but seems unable to combat effectively long-standing feelings of loss, grief, anger, guilt, and resentments that undermine its efforts in maintaining a positive and life-supportive energy flow. I do know, however, that a quality healer can significantly energize an ill person's body wisdom and can often facilitate dramatic and positive results.

Think of organs and systems of the body as having

imaginary energy tabs. These tabs eventually reflect all the things we eat and drink, all we experience physically, emotionally, and spiritually. These energy tabs act like mini-magnets in the etheric energy field, either attracting or repelling the energy of the body wisdom. When we're sick or depressed and upset, these tabs change to discourage energy from being drawn into specific parts of the body. Working on a person's energy field can encourage the body to regurgitate unpleasant memories, thus releasing negative energy to again attract the positive energy of the body wisdom.

## Love, Not Experience, Is the Essential Element

You choose to work on your friend or partner because you care about him or her and want to help. You don't need any previous experience. I've discovered that people have a natural capacity to help and heal each other and that, given a few simple directions, they can heighten their own intuitive senses and work effectively to encourage the swing toward health and emotional and spiritual well-being both for themselves and for others. Assume that you, too, will benefit from working with your friend. You will certainly want to share with your friend the ways in which you experience the energy generated from your combined work.

When we hold hands with or put our hands on another person, we may ask, "Am I doing it right? What if I make a mistake? What if I hurt the other person? What if the person thinks I'm strange for asking if I can help?" These are all very natural doubts; yet the healing benefits are well worth the effort to persevere. I remember the time many years ago when I had my gallbladder removed surgically in a large-city teaching hospital. Two people remain vivid in my memory for helping me through the pain and complications of my three-week stay.

One was a cleaning woman on the night shift and the other a nurse in the intensive care unit. Both spoke to me in soft and loving terms. Both were positive in their outlook on life and were comfortable touching me. Their way of being with me was immensely comforting. I often wished they could have some idea of how tremendously they helped me in ways that I'm sure they didn't even consider special. So consider the impact you have when you make your Love and energy available to another person.

## Preparations for Doing Your Healing Work

Some preparation is necessary before you begin to work with your friend or client. In my own work with clients, I've found it extremely helpful to pay attention to the following items:

1. Set aside enough time for your healing work. This can be thirty minutes or up to two hours. As you are working, you'll come to know intuitively when your friend or you have had enough. It's a good idea to begin with a short period, even fifteen minutes, and then gradually work up to a longer period, if agreeable to you both. The length of your healing time will depend on the health of your friend. People in a lot of pain find it unpleasant to sit in one position for very long. Remember to pay attention to your friend's body language as you are working. It will tell you if your friend is comfortable.

2. Find a quiet place where your friend can be worked on comfortably and not be interrupted by the telephone or other distraction.

3. Wash your hands in cold water before beginning. This helps clear your energy field and allows you to

approach your friend without carrying over negative energy.  Allow your own worries and fears to flow away with the water so that you can be present to act primarily as a channel, a conduit of universal and healing Love.

4. Have your friend get into a comfortable position by lying down, leaning back against a couch, leaning forward with head in hands and with lower back supported, or in any other position that allows you to work.  While the person can remain fully dressed, it will be easier for you to work when clothing is simple and soft so that your hands can move smoothly over the body.

5. Sit next to the person in any comfortable position so that your hands are free and so you can touch the person directly or work by keeping your hands several inches away from his or her body.  You are not expected to be an expert in body work, you are a friend who is learning a new way of helping someone you love and care about. Ask your friend to relax and to breathe normally.

6. Begin with a short inner centering.  I use a short prayer asking that I be guided to help in the best way and that my actions and intentions be those most appropriate to accomplish all that the Universe and my friend wish and need. You are now ready to begin your "hands-on" healing work.

## Hands-On Healing and Intuitive Listening

You will need both hands to move energy most effectively into and within your friend's body.  Place one hand on the person's solar plexus and the other at the small of the back, so your hands are approximately opposite each other. Usually, I close my eyes so that I can concentrate on what I'm feeling rather than on what might be attracted to my eyes. In a slow, clockwise motion, begin moving the hand over your friend's solar plexus in very small circles, gradually tracing larger and larger circles on the person's abdomen while moving your hands in a steady rhythm. Keep repeating this motion, working from the inside circle outward and then back inward to the small circle. After several minutes of this motion, allow your hands to move toward specific sites of pain or uneasiness or tension.

Another method I use to channel life-force energy to a person is to direct my movements to the feet or the palms of the hands. This creates another powerful connection through which the Universe's energy can pass to your friend.

With either the solar plexus method or the hands or feet method, close your eyes and allow your friend's body wisdom to guide your hands. Allow images and thoughts to flow freely into your awareness. At the same time, talk with your friend. Share with your friend what you are feeling or sensing. Restrict your conversation to affirming both the person's feelings, as he or she talks to you while you work, and to the positive nature of what you are sensing and attempting to do. Resist random negative speculation as to the extent, nature of, or future of the disease or trauma. What you may think is being offered in an offhand or speculative manner may easily be heard by your friend as a certainty.

As you put your hands over a specific organ or place on the body that feels painful to your friend or that you sense is in trauma, remember to keep a light touch, since when the person is in pain a small amount of pressure can feel intense. Ask for continual feedback from your friend on the nature of any relief that is felt, the intensity of your pressure, and what you are doing that the person likes or does not like.

Sometimes I hold my hands cupped together over a problem area. Sometimes I move them independently in sweeping or circular motions. Sometimes I move one hand to the person's chest or abdominal area and keep the other hand on the person's back. Making changes like this is where your own intuition comes in. You are responding in relationship to the energy you feel, so you are allowing your hands to move in ways that seem right, according to what you feel.

Even if you don't think you're feeling anything, allow your hands to move and glide in comforting ways. Any level of caring touch helps. The degree to which hands-on healing can help varies from mild relief of symptoms to a general re-ordering of the person's presence. You'll be able to notice these positive signs in the person: the eyes become clearer, the conversation is livelier, the individual's general energy level is heightened, a sense of well-being returns. And sometimes there will be a total remission of symptoms. Miracles in healing can and do happen.

## Your Responsibility as Healer

Every healer has a wide variety of experiences, from the removal of disease to merely a general and improved sense of well-being. Many factors are involved, not the least of which is your friend's depth of relationship with the Universe and understanding of the specific lessons involved in his or her spiritual learning. Your friend's relationship with the Universe may hold a disease or negative situation in place until he or she reaches a level of understanding at which release is possible.

Your task is not to second-guess the advice that your friend may need or the ways in which the Universe is present.

As a healer, you are merely the conduit, the avenue through which healing can happen. You are not responsible for either the level of healing or the seeming change or lack of change in your friend's physical condition. You are merely witnessing this person's life in a loving way, and you need to hold in your heart that the person receives well-intentioned energy through you no matter what change is physically or emotionally perceptible. Healing often takes place on the spiritual level, where we are unable to perceive it.

When a person is involved in energy work with another, the separations between people fall away, and people find themselves being honest and forthcoming, with insight into their lives, their fears, and their problems in ways that allow them to release built-up worries and fears. These thoughts are, of course, privileged information between you both, because by working on another, you establish a bond of trust that moves your relationship far beyond the normal friendship. The relationship should, therefore, be honored in appropriate ways.

## Gauging the Amount of Healing Work Required

In working to heal disease, we often wonder what it takes to heal a major disease versus a simple cold or emotional upset. The difference seems to lie in the quality and quantity of energy required. This means that if a person has the flu, working for several short periods can turn the tide toward healing. The same amount of work won't have the same effect on a more serious condition, because the body wisdom has been more seriously depressed and cut off from specific organs or body systems for a longer period of time.

The amount and quality of energy introduced into a person's body will vary. A big difference exists between turning on the current to a forty-watt light bulb in a large, dark warehouse and turning on a laser beam in a box. Energy commensurate with the "laser beam in a box" corresponds to the amount of time and quality of energy introduced into a person's body. If you are the person receiving the healing, you may find that it is helpful to have other members of your healing wheel working on you every few days. As you seek to turn the corner toward healing, you can sense a deep hunger for the energy your body needs.

We all have the capacity to help and heal each other. Giving and receiving Love, touching each other by mutual consent, is a very natural way we can help. Reaching out to touch another person in Love is always healing. Gently stroking a person's face, hair, hands, or feet also has a soothing effect on the body and the mind. Compassionate Love for another opens unimaginable doors to helping a person accentuate his or her own inner strength and courage.

In doing physical healing work, the placement of your hands on a person's body or the way you move your hands is less important than your loving intentions. Whenever you lay your hands on another person in Love, healing results on the most appropriate levels.

## Thoughts to Help You or Your Friend Heal

1. In order to heal the body and restore the energy of the body wisdom, give yourself continual encouragement in order to combat the opposite messages that you receive from others, and those that you give yourself, concerning the seriousness of your condition and any long-range prognosis.

2. To heal your body, all that is needed is to tip the scale in favor of the energy of your body wisdom. This

means that you don't need to worry about healing every tumor site, every place there is pain or trouble in your body. You are concerned simply with tipping the scale in favor of healing by allowing yourself to live within a spiritually and emotionally positive environment. Disease will always give way to the energy generated by your spirit through your prayers, invocations, and meditations. Disease cannot survive when the body wisdom is fully functioning.

When you are in pain, your own body doesn't have the energy necessary to keep the body wisdom functioning well. That is why creating an all-encompassing, pervasive personal environment of positive Love and acceptance of your lessons to be learned calls into action both the power of your own inner goodness— your self-worth—and the energy of the Universe.

3. All pain isn't symptomatic of deterioration. When a disease, dysfunction, or mis-alignment has existed in your life for period of time, repositioning the organs through energy work can be uncomfortable. Usually, a person can learn to distinguish between pain that is destructive and pain that is healing. All three aspects—your individual organs and systems, your thoughts, feelings, and beliefs, and your spiritual invocations, prayers, and healing energy work with others—contribute toward keeping the energy levels in your body high, thus keeping your body wisdom alert and active.

4. Focus your healing on one day at a time. That is all that is required. Resist the temptation to plan what the future will hold because you truly don't know.

5. If you are the one in need of healing, remember that a severe illness or emotional trauma requires an all-out

healing effort and is probably the biggest single challenge you will undertake in this lifetime. As you try to put the elements of your healing program together to relieve pain and to heal your body and your life, you walk a razor's edge. Sometimes you feel committed strongly to your healing and know you can be successful, and at other times you feel helpless and certain you will not get better. These ambiguous feelings tell you that you stand on this razor's edge. Your job is to bring yourself back to the affirmation that you are working with the Universe in the most appropriate ways and that energy, grace, and love are coming and will come to you in the most useful and productive ways for your life.

6. Sometimes, when you need healing, getting out of bed and beginning the day can seem like an overwhelming task. Pretend that you can do it. Say to yourself, "I can do this," disregarding the conflicting messages that tell you that of course you can't. The truth is that you can do a very great deal more than you think because you are drawing on the Universe's energy, not just the energy of your body. When your body tells you that it can't do something, that is because it is responding to its own level of energy. You, however, can also draw from your spirit and from your self-worth to add fresh energy to your life and your healing.

7. If you are working on healing yourself, make tapes of music that you find nurturing. Ask your friends to lend you books, audio and video tapes, or other materials that can help expand and enhance your spiritual understanding, your feelings of inspiration, and your positive growth. Also accept the offers from friends for food, errand-running, or rides. You are in charge of your own healing, and if you let others know the ways they can

help, they will. If you can afford to pay someone to do these things for you, that is even better. This allows you and your friends to keep the balance in your relationship on the basis of what they can give and choose to offer rather than what they must give.

8. Keep in mind that the God-force is an intangible presence, and that we often make a connection with this omnipotent force most easily through spiritual teachers or visual materials. Whatever symbols, pictures, poetry, or meaningful expressions of Divine Love are important to you, put them out in plain sight where you can enjoy and feel encouraged by them.

9. Consider your emotional as well as your physical health. While we work to improve our physical health, we need to also be building our emotional energy. Our losses continue to drain our bodies' energy unless we are undertaking to heal our emotional discontent simultaneously with strengthening the energy of our body wisdom.

10. Select and use a healing coach. When we are in pain we are not always capable of re-activating our body wisdom in the ways that are essential for a return to health. Thus it is vitally important to work with a healing coach and others in your healing wheel who can augment your own energy for healing. Remember that your primary job is to manage and direct your own healing and the energy of your body wisdom toward your own greatest good.

## Sharing Energy with Others

Working with others by placing our hands on another, whether with a casual touch or a touch with specific intent, is one of the most beautiful and meaningful ways we open ourselves up to the unknown Universe. We are trusting that we are all trying to grow and that our intention is to be of value and service to each other and to this life that we share. This touching process generates healing energy that helps restore a sense of well-being, of calling forth our own Love for ourselves and others.

From the personal standpoint of the healer, this means that you are allowing your own Love to invite the Love and total presence of the God-force to flow through your hands and thoughts into another person to reduce pain, to heal trauma, disease, and dysfunction, and to balance this person's total spiritual, emotional, and physical energy fields. Laying your hands on another person is an ancient healing practice that has been honored through the ages for bringing relief and joy to both the giver and receiver. Dolores Krieger in her book *Therapeutic Touch: How to Use Your Hands* was the first contemporary health-care practitioner to present a philosophy for healing, called "therapeutic touch," based on the ancient laying on of hands. Her work with the healer, clairvoyant Dora Kunz, has taught many thousands of people around the world an effective and meaningful technique for healing with their hands.[2]

The thought that whenever you lovingly place your hands on another person, a healing takes place on the most appropriate levels, is a powerful thought to contemplate. Whether the hands belong to a mother holding a crying child, a husband soothing his invalid wife, a nurse tenderly stroking a patient in pain, we as human beings have the capacity to do that which is basic to our natures—heal another person with our hands.

# NOTES

1.  Meredith Lady Young, *Agartha: A Journey to the Stars* (Walpole, NH: Stillpoint, 1984).

2.  Dolores Krieger, *Therapeutic Touch: How to Use Your Hands to Help Heal* (New York, NY: Prentice Hall, 1979).

# 12 Synthesizing the Energies of Body, Mind, and Spirit

*Choosing mind over matter really means finding spirit within life.*

We tend to separate our spiritual work from our everyday living. When we are in our "spiritual mode" we think spiritually: we meditate, work on our inner issues, seek balance in specific ways. When we are in our "other than spiritual mode," which is most of the day, we often override the inner voice of our spiritual energy, figuring that our time in meditation compensates for those other parts of our days and lives that are obviously imbalanced. This "drop-in-the-bucket" spiritual effort doesn't do very much to dent the enormous challenges we face in healing and recovering.

Today we can no longer separate our spiritual work from the rest of our living choices that carry over into our careers and daily jobs, our partnerships and friendships, and all the circumstances and people who figure the most prominently in our lives. Why? Because every one of these choices contribute in such important ways to our total health. For this reason we need a more complete perspective for using spiritual energy in life healing.

The stronger we become spiritually, the more significant (and in some sense the more obvious) are  misalignments in our lives. All aspects of our lives need to flow smoothly from our spiritual core. This doesn't mean we'll correct our imbalances overnight, but through awareness of those problem places and through working openly with those people with whom we have issues and those we draw comfort from, we build inner power and stem our energy leaks. When we hide from the fact that we have problem situations and bury our true feelings and spiritual initiatives, pretending that they don't matter, then we lose power.

## Spiritual Energy and Lifestyle Choices

The quality of our days is critical to our immediate and long-term healing and the contentment and joy of our living. Two factors are worth discussing here in order for each of us to ascertain the lasting lifestyle changes that we need to initiate.

In Chapter Three I identified the six spiritual energy influences of Love, and for each influence I listed the balanced emotional responses, those emotional responses that are energy leaks, and the systems and parts of our physical bodies that are at risk. Now, let's consider the specific spiritual lesson underlying each spiritual influence so that we can better understand our responsibility for living all day long in "a spiritual mode," for making appropriate lifestyle choices. I've written the spiritual lessons as invocations or affirmations because we can use these thoughts in our daily meditation work to heal the aspects of spiritual imbalance we've identified. I've also listed the lifestyle challenges that we need to address in each of the six spiritual energy influences as we seek to restore spiritual balance to our lives.

## Spiritual Lesson #1: Reflection

*I am willing to risk sharing my true self with others, because I believe in my own self-worth and my capacity to love myself and others. I am unafraid to try new and different things, because I accept that I will have ample chances in this and other lifetimes to respond to my challenges in a wide variety of ways.*

What does this knowledge of our eternal life mean at the lifestyle level? What choices do we make or not make as a result of accepting this spiritual truth? Let's consider the riddle of the "God mythology" in helping us explore our beliefs surrounding our immortality.

God is like a tiger. Sometimes we sense the ferociousness, other times the gentleness. Natives who live near jungles where tigers live have many a story to tell. These stories are no doubt exaggerated in the telling, and the fearsomeness and cunning of the tiger and the chase take on mythical proportions. God's mythical proportions can also scare us away from finding the Creator that is real for us and the beliefs that are essential to our growth. Much like the tiger, God is probably different for each of us depending on the context of our meeting Him, Her, or It in the dark of night or morning mist, stalking prey or nursing young.

Many people seem perfectly content to live without aspiring to discover or learn about the loftier realms of Divinity. Why should we make the effort to understand or even pray to a God-force when those who we trust to know tell us we can never understand this force? The new spiritual energy of the twenty-first century is challenging us to establish our own personal relationship with God and to move through our ambivalences, because this on-the-fence position holds no power personally or globally. We are in need of learning the ways to truly live in the energy of Love, with wisdom, independence, freedom, choice, and opportunity—all the qualities that are essential for a free society and a balanced, healthy world. Our relationship with God, the tiger, thus becomes truly significant.

We need a personal relationship with God if for no other reason than we need to know in what ways we fit with life and death and eternity. Even if some of us give God clothes and feelings that seem more appropriate to humankind than to the omnipotent Creator, nothing is lost as long as our image of God is based on Love—the kind of Love that encourages growth and expects each of us to pull our fair share of the load in this life.

The intricacies and mysteries of birth and death and all that lies in between can no longer be chalked up to pure chance. We see too much that is beyond rational explanation; too many scientific premises are being shattered as the simple on-going march of time shows us more and more of the truth about the relationship between the physical and nonphysical universes. The more we learn about truth, the more we want to learn, and the more we find there is to learn.

Life and the God-source are infinite, so it seems most appropriate to accept that we are part of a system that we may never fully understand as long as we are in physical form. The fact that we don't fully understand God does not negate the existence of a God-source. We see evidence of God everywhere we look, at every moment of every day. And the many faces of Love that we see are not always obviously soft, gentle, and accepting; much of the Love we experience forces us to grow and change in ways we are reluctant to accept because they hurt.

When we see evidence of God everywhere, we also see what we call evil. Evil seems to be the lack of "the light of the God-source." This means that *evil* is a name we give to represent those actions that are initiated apart from a loving intent. We are given pause to consider that evil doesn't manifest itself only in ruthless murders but is also present in any thought or action not originating from universal Love.

The existence of evil need not hinder our search for God. In searching for a personal relationship with God, we are approaching God, the Tiger, as the unknowable source of all things, all life, and all experience. We can learn of God each in our own way when we realize that trying to know God will provide us with different views and different experiences. Together, all our truths probably contain the reality of God.

We want to know God personally because we want to understand the mystery that we are living. We are drawn and driven by the uncertainty of life and the vastly different qualities we experience of Love and hate, wisdom and greed, selflessness and egotism. We are on our own search for God the Tiger, and the ways in which we encounter this spectacular force will lead us toward a greater truth and appreciation for all of life.

*Lifestyle Challenges for Using the Energy of Reflection*
- Prioritize your spiritual work.
- Give yourself a beautiful and meaningful place to meditate, pray, or sit quietly, even if you merely fix up a closet for this purpose.
- Fill your senses with the sights, sounds, and tactile sensations that give you pleasure and reaffirm your commitments to yourself.
- Eliminate "I can't meditate" from your vocabulary.
- Believe in yourself and your ability to find a meaningful and healing spiritual lifestyle.
- Be truthful in talking with others and in telling them what you really mean—tactfully, yet the whole truth.
- Trust that others will rise to the level of Love that you extend to them.

## Spiritual Lesson #2:  Partnership

*I am able to seek relationships that value my awakened spirit and my capacity to give and receive Love. I know that Love is the primary instrument of personal growth, and that my life will find meaning in relationships as I feel strengthened in my ability to be my own self and use the Love that I increasingly feel for myself, other people, and all other living things.*

We want to be loved; is that so bad?  Beyond the claims of dysfunction, misalignment, and victim consciousness lives a man or woman, boy or girl, in need of being loved.  Love can be sexual—but it is more.  Love can be emotional—but it can go further.  Love is respect for the journey through life. Love is the courage to honor the struggle as well as the accomplishment.  Love means that although we are part of the human dilemma, we can still see above the smog to the clean air of reverence for the spirit.

Of course we need Love, and we want a loving partner and loving friends. If we weren't designed this way, we wouldn't have so many problems getting into relationships, staying in them, and deciding when we must leave them. Love is energy, the most powerful energy in our lives. Love is within us even now and wants to find expression in our lives through partnership with others.

Partnership is important because it teaches us to share. Partnership helps us think about someone else's needs the same time we consider our own. Partnership is selfless and giving; it is also demanding and consuming. Partnership is the reflection of our capacity to love fully, with passion and endurance. And whether or not we are successful, whether or not we find pain in our search for Love, loving is a critical part of our spiritual growth.

Because Love is an energy, we build energy inside ourselves when we love. Our ability to love grows to where we can love even those we might have thought at one time were unlovable. Loving lets us see the sparkle in someone's eyes before we notice that the person has no legs. Love gives us enduring empathy for the person who is walled off in his or her own pain. For us to feel good, we give love that doesn't even need to be returned.

Partnerships—real, meaningful, lasting, loving partnerships with one specific person—are not always within our immediate reach. This requires that in addition to our seeking personal partnerships, we need additionally to also be seeking other kinds of friendships that allow us to love from our own awakened spirit and deepening spiritual values. Many around the world need Love, are dying from a lack of Love, would give anything to be loved. I believe our task is bigger than just seeking a personal partnership. The partnership model we are being called to fulfill extends way beyond our families and friends.

When we match our Love with those who most need it, we both win. We grow spiritually, and they grow spiritually, and all of us are better prepared to tackle life's struggles. Love heals beyond words and activates joy as does no other emotion. Even if we have personal partnerships, Love can grow beyond our spouses to planetary partnerships that include many others in need. We are not limited in the number of persons we can love. We can love far beyond what we may think. Love is self-perpetuating and will grow with the slightest encouragement.

Partnering is a model for living, working, and being together. Partnering is living with our spirits fully activated. Partnering is being with others in those ways that give satisfaction and allow personal growth. Our training and experience in personal partnership can be broadened so that we can become partners in new, more expansive ways and then can give Love through the ways that we are now learning. Partnering is a tool of spiritual and emotional change for our future, and those who are able to embrace a partnership model in all of their relationships are well positioned to facilitate positive global change.

### Lifestyle Challenges for Using the Energy of Partnership

- Choose friends and/or a partner who supports your efforts to grow emotionally and spiritually.
- Seek clarity in your relationships, and ask your current closest friend or partner how you and she or he can renew your relationship and help it grow to new levels.

- See those close to you as different each morning; rather than assuming you already know who they are, allow them to show you.
- Treat each other with respect, and encourage yourself and others to shoulder the responsibilities of personal growth.
- Practice loving those people who will never become close friends, whom you are afraid of or dislike, and whom you read or hear about but will never meet.

## Spiritual Lesson #3: Integration

*I am able to appreciate the spiritual, emotional, and physical aspects of my being and to improve communication between my spirit and my feelings, my feelings and my body, and my spirit and my body. I am able to do this to further an inner harmony that I realize is essential for my health and my appreciation of life.*

Inner harmony is difficult to find in our stressful lives and even more difficult to maintain as the basis for our living. Yet inner harmony is essential for stemming our energy leaks and allowing us to grow personally. Physical activity is meant to enhance our health by balancing our energy fields. Physical activity also awakens the inner emotional and spiritual levels of our beings that need realigning through mindful attention. Physical activity that we undertake as exercise encourages this process of inner harmony; so does energy body work, such as massage.

Exercise is, as we are aware, an effective means of reducing stress and encouraging health. Its purpose is not only to provide added oxygen to our system but also to exercise the body's frame and support structures. This

energy of Integration actually "supports our life" by balancing the energy of our body, mind, and spirit. If we feel
unsupported by life, we are lacking the inner harmony that
unifies our daily activities with our emotional needs and
feelings and our spiritual expectations.

The amount and type of exercise we do should, ideally,
match our emotional needs, our genuine interests, our body
types, and our lifestyle requirements. Exercise, even a straight
aerobic workout, should be mindful rather than mindless. This
means that the benefit to the body is increased when all three
energy fields (the etheric, the astral, and the spiritual) are awakened and stimulated through physical movement and are better
able to relate to each other and ultimately to support our lives.

In addition to straight exercise, we also need body work
like massage or any of the wide variety of hands-on energy-
balancing techniques. This kind of body work specifically
harmonizes and balances the body's energy. Massage is very
popular because it is a pleasant and easy way to receive the
benefit of energy movement. Massage is an ancient art and is
found in every culture on the planet. During massage we
place our hands on a loved one to offer reassurance and to
suggest acceptance, Love, and appreciation. We place our
hands on a fellow human to help remove pain, awaken
awareness, and induce relaxation and sleep. We stroke animals to reassure them and to help them heal.

When someone massages us, we experience a change in
our energy fields. We, like the other animals of the planet,
use our hands, our lips, our eyes, and our body language to
convey our joy and appreciation for this touch. What we are
truly grateful for is the sensation of inner balance and well-
being that is awakened through energy balancing.

Physical activity and realignment also awakens and releases
past memories still lodged in our tissues. Through this effort,

the energy of Integration heightens the energy of our spirits, giving us a more hopeful perspective for our future. When we enter into any physical activity or energy work involving the physical body, we are meant to experience movement and integration on the inner planes. Heightened feelings of well-being are common after exercise or body work because our energy is flowing freely, and we are more balanced.

When we have no physical movement in our lives, we also lose the emotional expansiveness that allows us to respond to others from a wide spectrum of feelings. Without physical movement we become frozen emotionally, self-pre-occupied, lacking in passion, and overwhelmed by much of our lives. We become uncomfortable when we are called on to deal with change and shifts in our feelings or in our philosophy of living. As our emotional well-being disappears, we come to believe we are being pushed past our limits by circumstances that in fact have engaged only our self-defined limited emotional boundaries.

Without the energy of Integration at work in our lives, we live out of touch with our real feelings and exhibit a lack of compassion for other people and living things. When we are without any form of physical movement, save walking around the house or to and from our cars, or sitting dutifully on our exercise bikes, we find it difficult to process stress, to enjoy love-making, to find inner joy, and to accept the challenges life has set for us.

Physical movement awakens our passion for living. When we feel passion for our partners, for a future for our children, for our lives and those of all other sentient creatures, then we are also awakening the passion for our worship of the Divine. Passion for life allows us to enjoy the fruits of our work and activity. When we lack passion, we are accepting our low level of internal vitality as normal.

The movement of all life is around us, and it is only as we appreciate our own capacity to feel, move, and respond to life that we find the ways we can contribute to the awakening passion for a different future. Our bodies seek balance through the energy of Integration, just as our planet seeks balance through change and realignment. Our passion for one awakens our passion for the other.

*Lifestyle Challenges for Using the Energy of Integration*
- Take time to exercise, and make it something you like to do.
- Have a massage or other type of body work on a regular basis.
- Pay attention when your physical body "talks" to you through pain; rather than always taking a pill to override the symptoms, first ask yourself and your body what hurts and why.
- Get to know your body, and discover the ways it wants to move and benefits from activity.
- Participate in physical, emotional, and spiritual activities that are meaningful to you.

## Spiritual Lesson #4: Alignment

*I am able to find my purpose for living by acknowledging my connection through Love to the God-source. This awakened relationship allows me to accept inevitable change and to initiate meaningful work and activities from an inner alignment with my spirit and the Divine.*

No one chooses intentionally to pursue meaningless work or participate in activities that are unrewarding. Yet we often find ourselves in jobs that we value for only the weekly paycheck, in careers that could be wonderful but aren't, or engaged in various ways of "earning our keep" that aren't giving us any inner satisfaction.

Meaningful life work doesn't emerge from the Puritan work ethic that tells us busyness, in and of itself, is the prize. Most of us have concluded that the "work until you drop" mentality is unsatisfying and self-defeating. I like to think of life work as more closely aligned with the original Shakers' philosophy of "hands to work and hearts to God," which suggests a relationship between what we do in life and our relationship with the God-force.

Every living thing needs to contribute in some meaningful way, through some essential work or activity, in order for the larger systems of Earth and universe to benefit and grow. In exchange for the opportunity of life, I believe we are required to give back our talents, skills, and wisdom to make the world a little bit better. If you feel unfulfilled in your work life, then consider whether or not the efforts of your spirit are reflected directly, indirectly, or in any way at all in your current job, career, and volunteer or community activities.

Our search for meaningful work is decidedly different from the ways we normally look for employment. Life work entails being in service to the Universe, and so our inner values are called to the fore to set the guidelines. The criteria by which we measure success in life work isn't tied to money, praise, accomplishment, recognition, or approval. It's tied to fulfilling that which we've incarnated to the Earth to contribute in this lifetime.

Once we've begun our spiritual work aware of our missions, those means of fulfilling our life work will find us. We need not be concerned initially with charting the "doing" part of our work. We do need, however, to affirm our potential and skill for helping or healing others and the Earth.

Meditation and quiet prayer are becoming essential practices to awaken the emotional and spiritual energy that can fill us internally. These times of listening and conversing with the Universe quell our personal fears and insecurities so that we can be of value without falling by the wayside at the first difficulty. In searching for our life work, our first order of business is to come to the Universe and ask to be guided in the process. This initial stage inevitably gives way to our opportunity to act from what we feel inside. When we trust that our relationship with the Universe is stronger than our need to control the outcome, we will be able to make wise choices for ourselves.

In taking one step at a time, from the quiet time of initial discovery through a period of strengthened awareness that our ensuing actions are appropriate, we are able to move ahead with our lives, ever cognizant of our spirits' intention and the work we are set on accomplishing. We determine the speed of our progress from consideration to action by recognizing the degree of Universal support we find for our initiatives. Where the spirit is willing, the specifics will always follow. Nothing stands in the way of our living our life work except our own inertia, fear, and uncertainty.

A real-life example comes to mind, one that epitomizes this shift from the lifestyle we are currently living to a life that reflects a different and more meaningful future. A woman in her late thirties was attending college in a nearby town. She had several children, had been in jail for drug and alcohol abuse, had been married several times to men with serious prison records, and had as her close friends the thugs in a notorious motorcycle gang. While serving time in jail this woman decided that she didn't want the life she was living and wanted a different future for herself and her children. Through all kinds of "coincidences" she found a way to complete her high-school equivalency requirements, be accepted into college, and get financial aid for her education. She talked openly about her fears and insecurities, but she talked the most about her experiences in prison that gave her time to think about who she really was and to discover that she felt "differently about herself on the inside."

The kind of work we do isn't important. What is significant is that we are doing it in harmony and alignment with our spirits' directive. We can find our life work only as we find our relationship with the God-force. As we take the time to work with the Universe, we will find the seeds of our life work in our everyday activities. Life work doesn't lie out in front of us barricaded with all sorts of hitches and glitches that can prevent us from fulfilling our mission. Nothing can prevent us from living our life work but ourselves.

If you are seeking your life work or are wondering whether what you are doing right now is the best thing for you, then take the time in your meditations to reflect on any activity of service, sharing, or participating with others in which you know you find meaning. These same ingredients of interaction that you find meaningful in your job, career, or community work will also be present in large measure in your life work.

Your life work often takes shape apart from what you've expected, needed, or felt you deserved. Meaningful life work is based on your genuine ability to parlay different elements of universal Love into a usable form for the benefit of a larger good. When you meditate, holding a genuine intention in your heart to know your path will help awaken the energy of Alignment and the power of your life work. The gift of this energy of Alignment is that once we realize that our life work is a natural extension of quiet inner work with the Universe, then we can stop struggling and begin to unfold into our real purpose for living.

*Lifestyle Challenges for the Energy of Alignment*
- Ask yourself if you feel that your work not only benefits you but also makes things better for others. If the answer is "no," then use meditation to reflect on what is missing and what you can do about it.
- Try to become more comfortable with change by altering small things in your office, in your home, or in your lifestyle. If you feel change frightens, upsets, or makes you irritable or angry, ask yourself in meditation for an explanation.
- Practice assuming that at this very minute your life work is unfolding for you. Affirm that it is already within your being and needs only your heart's permission and acceptance to surface with greater definition.
- Assume that the people and circumstances already in your life are part of your purpose and your learning. Find out what they have to teach you.

## Spiritual Lesson #5:  Rejuvenation

*I am able to participate with nature in understanding the cycles of my life. I accept these cycles in my life, knowing that they have a basis in Love. I acknowledge the times of struggle as well as joy, the times of birth as well as transition. I am willing to attend to my life work as well as I can, and then to relax, trusting that my efforts will bring successful completion*

Leisure time is an issue for everyone.  Should we take

the children and go to the mountains, or should we go to Disney World? Should we take the children at all, or should we go on that long-awaited get-away with just our partners? Or should we go off all by ourselves to find renewal? The many options we have to spend our discretionary time present us with important challenges. Some people like to go places where they can be waited on and relax in luxury. Others like to "rough it" and go camping or on wilderness expeditions. What are we looking for in our time away from our normal hectic life? One of the most important aspects of renewal from leisure time comes not from more stimulation of the human-made kind but from a more subtle and life-confirming stimulation that comes from nature.

Many people don't find sleeping in an open field, cooking over a camp fire, or rafting down a surging river to be fun. Other individuals are suburbanites or city-dwellers and are not excited by the pull of the wild. Yet I wonder if our lack of interest in experiencing nature comes from a lack of opportunity to learn to appreciate the different sort of challenges that being in nature offers.

Each of us can recount stories of meeting nature head-on that are extremely humorous because they reveal the extent to which most of us have lost the natural skill of finding joy and spiritual renewal in wilderness settings. We know how to navigate our way through a giant, sprawling shopping mall or weave our cars through crowded, winding inner-city streets to find an all-but-invisible parking space. But we've forgotten how to set our inner compass to walk unafraid into unspoiled lands and be nourished by nature. We shudder at sleeping unprotected under the stars for fear of being attacked by wild animals. We don't know how to "read" the land or how to regain our bearings when we wander off the beaten path.

Many people are quick to admit that when in nature they feel out of their element. Does this mean that we should accept this state of being, chalking it up to progress and our preference for humanly-devised entertainment and leisure activities over those offered by nature? Or should we make the effort to find nature where and when we can? Can nature teach us and help us live more meaningful and effective lives by understanding how to flow with the cycles of life and accepting that each cycle has purpose for our learning? How would our lives be richer if we worked in harmony with nature rather than only promoting our human agendas?

To answer these questions we need to decide what nature offers us that is essential. The ingredient that our lives most lack is random time, time spent without a goal, a drive, a purpose, a mission. Time spent merely observing life. Leisure-time activities that focus our attention and our responses offer us little in the way of rediscovering ourselves. The challenge of meaningful leisure time is to break out of the molds that we settle into and to rediscover a freshness about our lives. Just as snakes shed their skins, getting away from our normal work routines allows us to shed our purely human perspective for a period of time in order to claim those inner wild parts that have gotten lost or tamed.

As children we spent our leisure time in intriguing ways. We spent hours drawing pictures in the sand with a stick, kicking a ball through a mud puddle, or spitting watermelon seeds at our friends. Meaningful play, as any primary education teacher will attest, develops our creativity, our self-confidence, our ability to interact effectively and cooperatively with others. Creative play is as critical to adults as it is to children. Our leisure time can help us hold on to the inner parts of ourselves that are unexpressed in our normal living.

Leisure time in nature is absorbing because it permits us the freedom to participate in our own way without direction or constraint. Leisure time is also meaningful because we become part of something bigger than ourselves, and this feels safe and important. For that reason we like to sit and watch the waves. We are moved by dense and towering forests in which the trees seem to go up, up, up, out of sight, part of a system we believe in and hope will always protect us. We enjoy rediscovering that we are part of things without, for the moment, feeling our adult responsibility for the Earth's problems.

Standing in front of a bear's cage at the zoo isn't even remotely similar to standing on a bluff overlooking a rushing Arctic stream and watching a grizzly and her cubs sauntering down over the slippery rocks in search of salmon. It's important to feel awed by nature sometimes because this is the only way we'll work to protect the Earth's natural systems. We sometimes need to feel diminished by nature, experiencing life beyond our control or our total understanding—life that calls us to remember our shared kinship with the rest of nature. Seeing the great diversity of life in the wild gives us hope that a bigger, more immense reality exists beyond our humanness. We humans, for all our decisive actions that cut down, diminish, and eliminate aspects of the Earth's environment, are still children at heart, in need of the relationships that have all along given us pause to wonder.

### Lifestyle Challenges for the Energy of Rejuvenation

- Ask yourself, "If this were the last day of my life, in what ways would I want to spend it?"
- View being responsible as a positive thing, but avoid feeling responsible for everyone and everything.
- Remind yourself that what you accomplished today is

worth a great deal.
- Enjoy what comes to you naturally, and participate in nature with the same spontaneity.
- Teach your children to love wild things.
- Talk to yourself in the woods or other natural settings. And listen as well.

## Spiritual Lesson #6:  Nourishment

*I am able to find fulfillment in my life.  I am comfortable making the choices that feel satisfying to my body, my emotions, my intellect, and my spirit.  I am able to make my own choices regarding my lifestyle needs and to seek inner awareness when questioning the value of those things from which I seek nourishment.*

We human beings need nourishment at the physical, emotional, and spiritual levels.  We try ideally to nourish our bodies by choosing healthy and nutritious foods to keep our systems operating smoothly.  We accept that we are nourished emotionally by the Love we share with others.  And we know that the nutritional and energy components of food are important.  But especially critical is the spiritual component of what we choose to eat.

The spiritual aspects of nourishment come from the way that nourishment is produced.  In order for us to benefit spiritually from the foods we eat, or from the Love that we are given, we need to believe that the ways in which our foods are grown and the animals we eat for food are raised in alignment with our spiritual beliefs, and that the Love we are offered will nourish us spiritually.  Every time we experience a twinge of inner resistance to what we are eating or drinking, or the way we are giving or asking for Love, we can accept that something is out of alignment, and that we are receiving no real value from the exchange of food or feelings.

Foods that have life-force energy are the best for us. These are foods that come directly from the Earth and are not created synthetically. Foods that are eaten as soon as possible after picking retain the greatest amount of nourishment value. Foods that are grown organically, without pesticides or poisons, and that are unprocessed to retain essential vitamins and minerals, serve our systems in the best way.

Eating meat is an issue we will each need to decide for ourselves. The quantity of hormones, pesticides, and antibiotics found in most livestock is one barrier to safe meat-eating. The inhumane ways in which animals are raised and slaughtered means we have to deal with the fact that the flesh of these animals is filled with the emotional trauma and pain they experience as they are taken to slaughter. We would do well to remember that animals are conscious, sentient creatures that are not only an important part of the Earth's food chain but are also a meaningful part of our lives. Because we are trying to cleanse physical and emotional poisons from our bodies, it makes little sense to intentionally ingest foods and substances that are incompatible with our values and attitudes.

Humane and organic farming practices of all sorts are essential in order to raise and harvest food that is both appealing-looking and also filled with the vitality of a healthy growing and living environment. We become what we take into our bodies, and we are accountable for the ways in which we live and participate in the food-chain of our planet.[1]

Water and air quality are of concern to all citizens of the planet. We are unable to live without pure water to drink and clean air to breathe. At this point only a small fraction of the planet's fresh water supply is unpolluted, and the quality of air in many parts of the world is increasingly toxic to our bodies. The plethora of respiratory and immune deficiency diseases emerging are in part the result of our inattention to the quality of the Earth's natural resources and to our spiritual issues.

Living with the energy of Nourishment means questioning our choices at every turn. It means listening to our inner nudgings that tell us when we are eating in ways that grate against our spiritual initiatives. Healing happens both personally and globally when we live in harmony with the God-source and all living things. Because we tend to accept at face value the way foods look or are enticingly presented to us through advertisements, we may be oblivious to the fact that they are not nourishing us as we intend and need them to do.

Because there are so many people advising us about which foods and supplements we should be taking, making conscious food choices demands that we seriously weight for ourselves the spiritual components of these decisions. Most people know that they could benefit by eating less meat. For me, the issue of unnecessary suffering to our fellow creatures is the larger of the two issues. A friend recently summed his beliefs up quite poignantly when he said that he and his family didn't eat anything that could recognize its mother!

*Lifestyle Challenges for the Energy of Nourishment*
  • Ponder the ways that you are nourished not only by your choice of food and drink but also by the inten-

tions and beliefs that underlie these choices.

- Go for a walk in weather that is rainy, snowy, foggy, or windy, and notice the way you feel when you aren't rushed or mentally preoccupied.
- When you are outside, ask yourself, "What is the way I fit with this Earth?"
- When you look at the food you are about to eat, consider for a moment what you like about it; then, after you've eaten it, ask yourself if you still like the same things about it.
- Imagine a face on the animal or bird you are about to eat. Are you comfortable with this image? Does this animal or bird seem content with this exchange? If not, why not?

## Identifying Your Own Spiritual Energy Imbalances

The information presented in this book on the six spiritual energy influences of Love is meant not to be absorbed in one reading but to form a basis for continual spiritual work toward health and purposeful living.

Your healing work begins in earnest as you identify those underlying energy imbalances that have allowed you to get sick, stay in disease, or remain off-balance in any way. On the following pages I've listed the six spiritual energy influences, and for each influence, the following corresponding aspects: the effect of that energy influence felt by all living things, the spiritual lesson brought to the surface for our learning (stated as an affirmation), the emotional issues we are supposed to address, the physical body parts and systems that are at risk when this energy is unbalanced, and the lifestyle challenge/choices presented us by this energy influence.

To determine which of the six spiritual energy influences are the weakest in your life, first identify the physical
body parts and/or emotional imbalances that most closely
approximate those that are giving you trouble, and put a
check mark next to those categories. Next, identify those
lifestyle challenges that you recognize as being difficult for
you, and put a check mark next to those categories. Those
check marks, flag weaknesses of the energy of Love in your
life. Even if you marked only one of the physical, emotional, or lifestyle categories in any specific energy influence,
realize that the entire list of the corresponding aspects of
that energy influence require your attention.

If, for instance, you've had a heart attack, you would
locate "heart" in the category " Your Physical Body Parts
and Systems at Risk" under the "Energy of Partnership"
heading (spiritual influence #2) and place a check mark
next to it. This means that you are at risk for all the emotional and physical aspects of this energy influence, and the
spiritual lesson and lifestyle challenges stated under #2,
Partnership, are what you need to work on.

If, for another example, you know that you have a hard
time staying centered and accommodating change in your
life, then the emotional issues dealing with maintaining
inner balance relate to you. So place a check mark next to
the category entitled "Your Emotional Issues" under the
energy of Alignment (#4). This means that you are at risk
for all the emotional and physical aspects of this spiritual
energy influence, and the spiritual lesson and lifestyle challenges listed under this aspect of Love are what you need to
work on.

Take a few moments now to examine the charts on the
next several pages. Identify the physical body parts and/or
emotional issues that are giving you trouble, as well as the

lifestyle challenges/choices with which you are experiencing difficulty. The sequence in which the six spiritual energy influences are presented on the charts has a purpose that will be explained to you in the next chapter. Performing this exercise is important because in the process you will discover the underlying causes of many of your distresses, frustrations, fears, and anxieties, not to mention your physical disorders.

# Spiritual Energy Influence #1: Reflection

### Its Effect on All Living Things
All living things awaken eventually to the realization that they are aspects of Divine Love and thus live beyond any physical form.

### Its Spiritual Lesson for You
### (Stated as an Affirmation)
I am willing to risk sharing my true self with others because I believe in my own self-worth and my capacity to love myself and others. I am unafraid to try new and different things, because I accept that I will have ample opportunities in this and other lifetimes to respond to my challenges in a wide variety of ways.

### Your Emotional Issues
- Showing people your real needs and beliefs.
- Loving yourself.
- Trying new and different things, whether or not others agree or go along.
- Believing in your choices.
- Building faith in the God-force.
- Trusting that you are held in Love during and after physical life.

### Your Physical Body Parts & Systems at Risk

*Lymphatic/immune system*—spleen, lymphatic vessels, lymph

The immune system is made up of specialized cells, secreting substances called antibodies, that are custom-designed to disable the myriad of organisms that threaten health. Additionally, other chemicals circulate in the blood, ready to attack organisms that have been slated for destruction. Such diseases as cancer, AIDS, environmental and immune-deficiency diseases, and Epstein-Barr infection (mononucleosis) are all examples of diseases arising from an impaired immune system.

### Your Lifestyle Choices

- Prioritizing time for worship, such as in prayer or meditation.
- Incorporating spiritual practice into your everyday life and your speaking vocabulary.
- Joining with others in rituals and in celebration of your own Divine self, the Earth, and the God-force.
- Seeking knowledge and wisdom from those teachers who are in physical life and those who are in the spiritual realms.
- Honoring your spirit and its eternal relationship to the God-force.

# Spiritual Energy Influence #4:  Alignment

### *Its Effect on All Living Things*
All living things are encouraged to realize that the changes in their lives reflect essential changes of universal energy from the God-source, and that this energy is meant to help them clarify their own purpose for living.

### *Its Spiritual Lesson for You*
### *(Stated as an Affirmation)*
I am able to find my purpose for living by acknowledging my connection through Love to the God-source.  This awakened relationship allows me to accept inevitable change, and to initiate meaningful work and activities from an inner alignment with my spirit and the Divine.

### *Your Emotional Issues*
- Accommodating change in your life.
- Believing in your purpose for living.
- Acknowledging your own value and uniqueness.
- Accepting your right to a fulfilling life.
- Finding happiness through the clarification of your purpose.
- Accepting that your purpose grows from Divine Love.

### Physical Body Parts & Systems at Risk

- *Nervous System*—brain, spinal cord, ganglia, nerve fibers, and sensory and motor terminals
- *Endocrine System*—thyroid, parathyroid, pituitary, adrenals, portions of glands with ducts like Islets of Langerhans in the pancreas, portions of the ovaries and testes, and the pineal gland.

### Your Lifestyle Choices

- Using your time, talent, money, and effort on behalf of meaningful work that contributes to life in a positive way.
- Encouraging and supporting others as they change, and helping institute essential changes wherever you find that they are needed.
- Assessing your inner talents, joys, and skills in determining the type of work you want to pursue or to initiate where you already work.
- Making the effort to do what you feel you want or need to do, and accepting that the God-force will cooperate and mold your life in meaningful directions.

# Spiritual Energy Influence #2:  Partnership

***Its Effect on All Living Things***
All living things bond initially and continually with the God-force.  The spiritual energy blueprint for all living things is to eventually accept that Love is the primary component of bonding.  This suggests that all living things seek bonds to encourage spiritual development in addition to procreating or furthering of their kind.

***Its Spiritual Lesson for You***
***(Stated as an Affirmation)***
I am able to seek relationships that value an awakened spirit and the capacity to give and receive Love.  I know that Love is the primary instrument of personal growth and that my life will find meaning in relationships as I feel strengthened in my ability to be my own self and use the Love that I increasingly feel for myself, other people, and all other living things.

***Your Emotional Issues***
- Seeking a spiritual basis in relationships.
- Giving and receiving Love in an appropriate balance.
- Accepting that Love is the primary instrument of personal growth.
- Honoring the learning opportunities presented to you by your spirit.
- Accepting your spiritual guidance.
- Seeking guidance to direct your relationships and to glean the learning that is presented.

### Your Physical Body Parts & Systems at Risk

*Reproductive system*—in the male, testes, seminal vesicles, penis, urethra, prostate; in the female, ovaries, Fallopian tubes, uterus, vagina, vulva, and breasts.
*Circulatory system*—heart, blood vessels, and blood.

### Your Lifestyle Choices

- Choosing friends and/or a partner who supports your efforts to grow emotionally and spiritually.
- Changing or leaving relationships that prevent you from living the spiritual values based on Love and compassion that you deem essential for your growth.
- Teaching your children what you believe the spiritual values to be for marriage, partnership, friendships, and interactions with those who are strangers, but allowing for disagreement and discussion.
- Seeing each person you meet as a "partner" who also wishes to deepen his or her relationship to the Universe, and feeling confident in saying and doing what feels right to you because it is based on Love.
- Accepting others' comments, even disagreement, as a positive contribution to the furthering of your own study by causing you to question and refine your own beliefs.

# Spiritual Energy Influence #5: Rejuvenation

### Its Effect on All Living Things
All living things participate in cycles within physical
life that imitate the larger cycles of life and death.
These are spiritually-ordered, encouraging the alternation between periods of contraction or focused attention and those of rest and relaxation.

### Its Spiritual Lesson for You
### (Stated as an Affirmation)
I am able to participate with nature in understanding
the cycles of my life. I accept these cycles, such as joy
and struggle, birth and death, as natural cycles of all
life, knowing that they have a basis in Love. I am willing to attend to my life work as well as I can, and then
to relax, trusting that my efforts will bring successful
completion to my efforts.

### Your Emotional Issues
- Accepting that all aspects of your life move in
  cycles: from fear to Love, from loss to gain,
  from disease to health, and from life to transition.
- Acknowledging that your cycles are normal
  because they reflect the same cycles of change
  within nature and the God-system.
- Pursuing quality relaxation and accepting that it
  is as essential to your well-being as the times of
  focused attention.
- Finding that relaxation in natural settings offers
  a critical aspect of reflection and rejuvenation
  unavailable through human-made facilities.

### Your Physical Body Parts & Systems at Risk

*Respiratory system*—nose, pharynx, larynx, trachea, bronchi, and lungs.

*Excretory system*—kidneys, ureters, bladder, urethra, and skin.

### Your Lifestyle Choices

- Seeing nature as the ultimate teacher of cycles, and so participating in nature by hiking, camping, or spending time in parks, forests, nature preserves, and the wild places near you.
- Bringing nature into your home through living plants, terrariums, greenhouses, caring for pets and learning their ways of being.
- Measuring your "workaholic" tendencies against the value of time spent considering the joy and blessings you have in your life as well as your relationship to life that is so fleeting.
- Helping with the care and protection of wild birds and animals, as well as observing or photographing them in their natural settings.

# Spiritual Energy Influence #3:  Integration

### *Its Effect on All Living Things*
All living things have an inner integrity that is composed of spirit within a physical form.  Each living system will come to know and honor its unique presence
and function through experiences within specific living
environments.

### *Its Spiritual Lesson for You*
### *(Stated as an Affirmation)*
I am able to appreciate the spiritual, emotional, and
physical aspects of my being and to improve communication between my spirit and my feelings, my feelings
and my body, and my spirit and my body.  I am able to
do this to further an inner harmony that I realize is
essential for my health and my appreciation of life.

### *Your Emotional Issues*
- Creating a dialogue among your spirit, emotions, and thoughts to create a single inner
  theme or balance.
- Learning to use your intuition to help you
  determine what your physical body is lacking.
- Accepting that you have value, and learning to
  wait for the "second-response" emotions that
  help you act in Love.
- Allowing your spirit to show you its full potential for Love and the ways to apply this to the
  inner physical and emotional places where you
  hurt.

### *Your Physical Body Parts at Risk*

*Sensory parts*—eyes, ears, and nose. (Mouth and
tongue, while also sensory parts of the body, are
listed under #6, Nourishment)
*Skeletal system*—bones and connective tissues
*Muscular system*—muscles
*Tissues*—cells and groups of cells arranged as tissues
(excludes the tissues of specific organs).

### *Your Lifestyle Choices*

- Pursuing meaningful exercise and activities that
harmonize the physical body and furthers your
inner harmony.
- Accepting that massage and energy work on
your body is an essential aspect of maintaining
inner harmony and balance.
- Identifying your own self-worth, and trying to
respond to the people and situations in your life
from this inner place of self-validation.

# Spiritual Energy of #6: Nourishment

---

### *Its Effect on All Living Things*

All living things eventually accept that they are nourished most significantly by Love. While all living elements need many kinds of nourishment, only nourishment that is aligned with the spiritual intention of perpetuating Love is able to fully heal or sustain life.

### *Its Spiritual Lesson for You (Stated as an Affirmation)*

I am able to find fulfillment in my life. I am comfortable making the choices that feel satisfying to my body, my emotions, my intellect, and my spirit. I am able to make my own choices regarding my lifestyle needs and to seek inner awareness when questioning the value of those things from which I seek nourishment.

### *Your Emotional Issues*

- Finding the fulfillment that is already present in your current life.
- Making choices for your emotional, mental, and physical satisfaction that are aligned with your spiritual values.
- Seeking your own inner guidance when questioning the value of the things others tell you are good for you.
- Changing what you are capable of changing immediately, in order to align your spiritual beliefs and initiatives with your actions, and accepting that the time-frame for these changes is between you and the God-force.

### Your Physical Body Parts at Risk

*Digestive system*—alimentary canal, including
mouth, tongue, salivary glands and teeth,
pharynx, esophagus, stomach, small and large
intestines, pancreas, and liver.

### Your Lifestyle Choices

- Choosing the lifestyle that you feel is aligned
  with your spiritual beliefs.
- Accepting foods that are derived from healthy
  and organic harvesting practices, and if animals
  are eaten, choosing those that are raised and
  slaughtered humanely.
- Improving the quality of the natural resources
  you use by giving back more than you take and
  conserving Earth's resources so that there will
  be enough to go around.
- Realizing that your physical body is a reflection
  of the harmony or lack of harmony found
  presently between your spirit and the physical
  and emotional materials, thoughts, and feelings
  that you consume and absorb daily.

## Shifting Your Living Environment

Healing requires effort and thought. If you are willing to prioritize your relationship with your own spirit because you believe that you are making a transformative step in your life, you will begin to change dramatically and to find the God-source in ways you never imagined. Your life is one unbreakable whole, so you are healing more than your immediate disease or problem; you are seeking to heal your life. If you have trouble understanding this model of life-healing, keep trying. Don't give up because you think it's too involved or that you won't be able to figure it out. How much do you want your life to be different? Are you willing to work at it?

Our challenge is always to move through the barriers set up by our personalities. Our apathy, sense of self-defeat, or hopelessness comes not from our spirit or the God-source but from our human perspective that lives at the rational personality level. Lifestyle healing requires that all our inner and outer energies mesh. Whatever we are doing that doesn't fit with the way we think and feel creates an energy leak.

After we move out of the crisis mode of healing, we can move more into prevention, by accessing our hurts and pains initially as spiritual imbalances and by dealing with them more thoroughly at the times they occur rather than allowing them to become buried and imbedded in our psyches.

Each aspect of our lives, every single incident and encounter, and every thought, feeling, attitude, and belief affects our health. We cannot separate one part of our lives from the others. When we are in spiritual crisis, we are faced with the need to make decisions for ourselves even before we are sure we are making the right ones. No matter, we begin where we can, with whatever we can accept and absorb. Every effort counts and makes a difference.

You are your own best guide in using your intuition to

judge the quality of the choices you are making for your own healing and well-being. While the physical aspects of your healing and recovery are significant, remember that you are involved primarily in shifting the emphasis in your total living environment toward a spiritual perspective. This means that you are a unique and beautiful aspect of creation, and from your own spirit flows the insight, truth, and wisdom to reshape your future totally. Whether you choose a holistic or more traditional path to healing isn't the important thing; what makes the biggest difference in your healing is your belief in your chosen course of action and the force of your spirit to support this action. Your own attitude is the mainstay to a synthesized energy field and meaningful path to healing.

## NOTES

1. John Robbins, *Diet for a New America* (Walpole, NH: Stillpoint Publishing, 1987).

# 13 The Six Spiritual Energy Influences Come into Your Life in Paired Relationships

*Life is not what it seems, it is so much more!*

Up until now we've talked about each of the six spiritual energy influences primarily as distinct influences, which they are. Yet they also have important paired relationships. Understanding these relationships offers you additional insights for plugging the energy leaks that cause imbalance. I've called the process of synthesizing body, mind, and spirit energies for each of the six aspects of spiritual energy "a model for life healing."

As I worked with clients using this life healing model, I discovered that when a person had a major identifiable imbalance in one of the six influences, the energy influence

**Figure 3:**
**The Six Spiritual Influences of Love and**
**Their Paired Relationships**

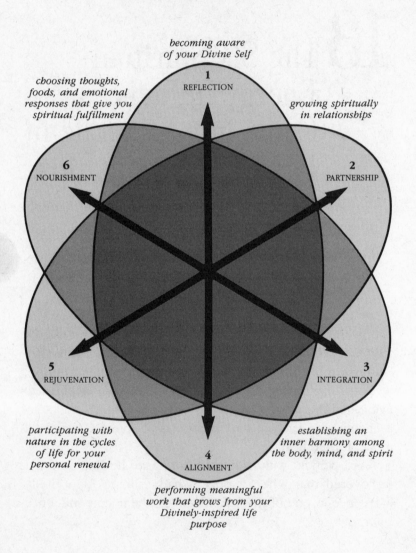

lying directly opposite it in my model was also greatly affected. This second energy aspect of all the other influences has the most direct relationship with the initial energy influence. That second energy aspect is such a specific complement so closely related to the first as to require pairing with it. So my model for life healing is arranged to demonstrate the paired relationships among the six spiritual energy influences.

As you match your own life's physical and emotional energy leaks against this model for life healing, you'll be intrigued to discover the extent of influence that spiritual energy maintains in your life. You'll find meaningful answers to many of the physical and emotional imbalances you've been merely accepting and living with.

Looking at Figure 3, "The Six Spiritual Energy Influences of Love and Their Paired Relationships," you'll see indicated the following relationships between two of the six spiritual energy influences, or aspects of the energy of Love:

- #1, Reflection (becoming aware of your Divine self), pairs off with #4, Alignment (performing meaningful work that grows from your Divinely-inspired life purpose).
- #2, Partnership (growing spiritually in relationships), pairs off with #5, Rejuvenation (participating with nature in the cycles of life to be renewed as well as stimulated).
- #3, Integration (establishing an inner harmony among the body, mind, and spirit), is paired off with #6, Nourishment (choosing thoughts, foods, and emotional responses that give you spiritual fulfillment).

Let's explore each of these paired relationships to understand the ways each relates to the other and the effect that imbalance in one specific energy influence has upon its paired mate.

## Balancing Reflection (God-awareness) with Alignment (meaningful work/life purpose)

The paired relationship between the energy influences of #1, Reflection, and #4, Alignment, as identified in Figure 3 might be called the "spirit in action bond," because it involves both our personal relationship with God and our meaningful life work on behalf of the Universe.

### When Your Dominant Imbalance is in #1, Reflection

The energy of Reflection awakens our relationship to the God-force and, through our own initiatives, teaches us perceptual skills in relating to the Divine. Any imbalance in this aspect tells us that we and the God-force have yet to find a comfortable working partnership. We may have trouble praying or meditating, or we may feel inadequate or disconnected from God even though we go through the motions of worship. We may have undergone oppressive experiences through prior religious training that we felt was dogmatic and constraining and often just unfulfilling. We may have felt that a personal relationship with God was irrelevant or unattainable, and so we've channeled our search for spiritual awareness into other means of fulfillment.

Because of its pairing with the energy of Alignment, the energy of Reflection affects our life purpose, too. We will find it difficult to identify, create, or sustain the work of our life purpose in a truly satisfying manner. Because life purpose arises from our spiritual work and personal discovery, we are obliged to open the door to personal spiritual awareness before we will find and be able to create or maintain purposeful life work.

Healing this imbalance lies in accepting that the basis

for our present spiritual crisis is basically spiritual and requires us to take our spiritual search seriously. Beginning to glean information, ideas, questions, insights, and perceptions from our spirits will help us better appreciate the role spirit plays in our lives. It is our spirits that originate our creativity and our personality that displays this insight most appropriately. All too often, our personalities assume the role of creative director in our lives and alter, contour, disrupt, and misrepresent the purpose and messages our spirits wish to bring into our lives.

### When Your Dominant Imbalance is in #4, Alignment

The energy of Alignment helps us accept our changing living environment and continue to stay focused on our life purpose and our work for the Universe. If we are imbalanced in this aspect, even though we may perceive and even be engaged in our life work, it will feel incomplete and inadequate to our expectations. We'll know something important is missing because this work is not sustaining us in ways that we want and need. Our life work or our ability to accomplish it the way we might want remains out of our reach.

In order to heal this imbalance of Alignment we will need to awaken our spiritual beliefs. In all likelihood we either already know a great deal about spirituality and feel we are too advanced to return to basics to see what else needs to be learned, or we are totally resistant to the idea of a spiritual framework for our life work. Either way, the spiritual dimension rules meaningful life work, and so if we want our purpose for this life to come into full focus and satisfy our needs rather than only the needs of others, then this is the avenue that requires re-opening or re-discovering.

## Balancing Partnership (growing spiritually in relationships) with Rejuvenation (cycles of our lives/nature as our teacher)

The paired relationship of #2, Partnership, and #5, Rejuvenation, as shown in Figure 3, could be referred to as the "relationship bond." This pair of energies affects our relationships with partner, family, friends, and community as well as with the natural world.

### When Your Dominant Imbalance is in #2, Partnership

The energy of Partnership oversees the spiritual quality of our relationships. Imbalance in this aspect suggests that our personal-partner relationship or close friendships are lacking in some significant way. We are aware that we want and need these relationships to be more nurturing and meaningful. We may have a history of poor partnerships, or we may be frustrated in our ability to find the right person or create the close network of spiritually-ordered friendships that we want. Healing occurs as we willingly acknowledge the spiritual components essential to our relationships and allow others to understand the importance we place on personal spiritual work.

A dominant imbalance in Partnership energy, because of its relationship with Rejuvenation, suggests that we have difficulty relating to the natural world in spiritual terms. When we are unable or unwilling to bring a spiritual presence into our everyday relationships, we are also unable or unwilling to accept comfort from the natural world in the way of spiritual renewal. We tend to separate nature from the spiritual dimension, seeing nature as a meaningful living environment but not in any terms that lead us to consider our own spirituality. The opportunity to heal and support our relationships can be substantially enhanced by allowing nature to become our spiritual teacher.

Many times, people who are imbalanced in the energy of Partnership have trouble initially accepting a meaningful relationship with the God-source and are more comfortable being led to this relationship through the intricacies and beauty found in the natural world.

*When Your Dominant Imbalance is in #5, Rejuvenation*
The energy of Rejuvenation calls into play our ability to live within the physical as well as spiritual cycles of our lives. We know, for instance, that when we eat we also need to eliminate the unneeded remains of what we've eaten. We feel urged to make love at some times and to rest at others. We need to sleep so that later we are awake to go about the business of our daily activities. We have emotional cycles that involve giving Love and receiving Love, asserting our beliefs and accepting those of others. We are also required to respond to the larger spiritual cycles of inception, growth, maturation, and transition, just as all living things do. When we are imbalanced in this energy of Rejuvenation, we see and respond only to part of the cycles of our lives. We selectively accept the psychological and physical aspects of change and personal growth but without finding the spiritual source from which all of this springs.

A dominant imbalance in Rejuvenation energy, because of its paired relationship with Partnership, tells us that we also create relationships that are incomplete. We tend to create relationships that are strong in the physical and perhaps even emotional arenas but short in the spiritual. We may have adopted patterns of living that deny our own greatest inner truths and needs. Healing comes from accepting the full spectrum of nature's cycles and using our time in, and love of, nature to allow ourselves to be led further into our spiritual convictions. We will then discover meaningful spiritual qualities emerging in our relationships as well.

## Balancing Integration (inner harmony of body, mind, and spirit) with Nourishment (fulfillment/life acceptance).

As depicted in Figure 3, the energy of #3, Integration, has a paired relationship with #6, Nourishment. This paired set might be called the "synthesis bond" because this energy involves finding and maintaining our own inner balance and then finding a lifestyle balance that is supported by all our personal and lifestyle choices and needs.

### When Your Dominant Imbalance is in #3, Integration

The energy of Integration influences our ability to create and maintain inner balance. It gives us the ability to harmonize the needs and requirements of our bodies, minds, and spirits by allowing for an inner dialogue that keeps each aspect aligned with the others. When we are imbalanced in the energy of Integration, we continually lose our sense of inner balance and centeredness. We struggle to maintain our own center and self-worth, and we find we are easily pushed and pulled by other people's wants, needs, likes, dislikes, and requirements of us.

Healing this imbalance of the energy of Integration requires us to discover and live from our own self-worth and inner goodness. We must first find our personal value in order to allow it to become the steadying force in our lives. As we find personal value we also awaken self-love that keeps us aligned even when the world dismisses our needs or when we are seemingly unable to create what we want or need most immediately.

A dominant imbalance in the energy of Integration,

because of its paired relationship with Nourishment, means that we have trouble making appropriate lifestyle choices that reflect our spiritual beliefs. We tend to be persuaded to change jobs, to change friendship and partners, to change or ignore living and eating habits even while we may secretly question our own actions. We try to fix our lives according to the criteria of others. Healing requires our returning to our own self-worth and self-love and allowing this energy to become the primary influence in our lifestyle choices.

### When Your Dominant Imbalance is in #6, Nourishment

The energy of Nourishment determines our ability to support and nurture our lives on all levels. When we are imbalanced in this energy we feel unsupported by our lives. We feel that life has let us down, we have failed, or we are lacking in the necessary skill, talent, education, or monetary resources required to be successful. Healing in this aspect means that we accept that success and support of life come first from a spiritual set of criteria based on service and initiating Love into life. Our challenge is to accept the power and integrity of our spiritual nourishment and the ways that we find meaning in supporting Love in our own lives. From this acceptance flows the ability to create meaningful lifestyle choices based on our full range of beliefs, feelings, and needs.

Because of Nourishment's pairing with Integration, when we have an imbalance in the energy of Nourishment it means that we also have work to do with the energy of Integration. With an imbalance in Nourishment, our lack of equanimity in our lifestyle choices causes us to remain fragmented in our own inner balance. We continually make choices that reinforce external power rather than internal power, and we always have reasons for being unable to make the choices that we say we want to make. Healing at the level of Nourishment means that we are able to choose the ways of eating, drinking, living, working, and finding support for our lives that lead us to inner harmony and centeredness.

## You Can Heal through Simple Awareness

If all these explanations have your head spinning, then recognize that you are considering life healing even though you feel that your most obvious problem is physical or emotional. Healing requires an overhaul of your life and the intricate ways in which all the pieces and energies fit into your life. You cannot fix just one pain or trouble and expect it to make the difference you want. Any serious effort to heal will inevitably take you deeply into the very questions of purpose, self-worth, and Love that this book addresses.

By taking one piece of this life-healing model to work with until you understand it thoroughly, you'll keep from becoming overwhelmed, and you will find questions, thoughts, and personal discoveries to explore further in your daily meditations. As you remember that your healing is a life-long process, you will be able to more readily accept the spiritual adventure that you've begun.

Many benefits can be forthcoming from your work, and the greatest of these is self-discovery. It is in acknowledging the all-powerful and pervasive influence that spiritual energy plays in your life that you are able to accept change as positive. As you find your spiritual footing you will be able to experience life from a place of inner confidence that brings you greater happiness and meaning. In working with this model of life healing you will no doubt come to value and appreciate your own life and its potential and the opportunities that are all around you. Addressing healing at the level of your spiritual energy strengthens your bond with the God-source and gives you the capacity to use Love as the means of healing your own life, the lives of those you love, and the Earth and her creatures.

# 14 Seeking Your Vision for The Future

*A vision is a story of sorts, a story relating to the value of your life, the reason you're on the Earth, and what it all means.*

Healing at both the personal and the planetary levels begins with our vision for the future. We are learning that initiatives for change lie within us and that, if we want to change our lives for the better and restore health to our planetary systems, we must give them the power of our voices and commitment. We must have a vision. Spiritual crisis is calling us to reorder our living patterns because we've been living without a vision for our own future. Groups, too, need a vision. The governments of the world's widely divergent populations have only recently begun to consider the building of a mutually supportive, peaceful, and sustainable world—a collective vision.

# Visions Are Humanity's Guideposts

Visions are not new. People have always had visions, although many times they weren't sure what to call them or what they meant. A vision is a story of sorts that is pulled from deep within us. It suggests ways we can rise to new levels of Love for both ourselves and others. Visions are humanity's guideposts for the ways we can collectively and individually walk the "higher road." When Martin Luther King called out to people everywhere, saying, "I have a dream," he was speaking for all of humanity, claiming equality for all peoples. When John F. Kennedy spoke at his inauguration, saying, "Ask not what your country can do for you, ask what you can do for your country," he was speaking to people's hearts and emotions rather than their intellects, inspiring them to reach beyond their normal acculturated responses. These men had visions of what the future could be.

We know that we want our lives and the lives of our children to be different. An old man who has lived for many years on the streets of New York City was interviewed one afternoon, and with tears in his eyes he said, "I've lived my life—I'm old, and no one wants me, and that's okay— but what about our children, what about our children?" This man has a vision of the future.

A vision of a better life involves healing this life. Healing has so many implications. Healing ourselves involves helping those around us to heal; healing ourselves means helping our world to heal. When we strive to heal ourselves we create humanity's vision for a brighter future. If this task sounds too enormous and difficult, then we must ask ourselves what the alternatives are.

In seeking to answer some of life's most challenging philosophical questions we often get bogged down in the rational and miss the true intention of inspiration, which is to unleash our own innate capabilities to create life in the image of Love. Until we willingly accept that visions do happen, are important to seek, are the basis for shared spiritual experience, we continue "to lead lives of quiet desperation."

I'm reminded of a well-loved old Sydney Poitier film, *Lilies of the Field*, in which Poitier's character gives a blind girl her first glass of pineapple juice. It's an astounding sensory experience for her, and additionally shows her, quite poignantly, the extent of life that she has missed. The spiritual search for our vision is this way. Until we find it or a part of it, we never know what we've been missing.

A vision is a manifested conversation between you and the God-Source. It is you and eternity conversing as to what you are to be giving your time, Love, attention, and effort to in this lifetime. How can you not want to know what your life is directed toward accomplishing?

## Finding Your Own Vision

There are many paths to finding our visions. They all involve confronting our personal dark night of the soul and that of humanity: enduring, withstanding, and accepting physical and emotional pain and duress in order to see ourselves more clearly in the image of the Divine. This is the path we all walk today and seek to emerge from. Great teachers of the past walked this path. Jesus Christ wandered in the desert for forty days and forty nights; Buddha sat under the Tree of Knowledge awaiting enlightenment; Gandhi was, several times in his life, prepared to fast unto the death in order to bring people together. The difference between these great teachers/mystics and ourselves is that they had a greater degree of spiritual balance and were thus able to hold an intention and manifest physical change through their beliefs. As a result, they sought union with the God-force and through this union were able to give clout to their personal initiatives.

A vision is given to us to make the most of the spiritual energy we already have and to develop in ways that augment this energy. Opportunities for using our spirits' energy abound every day. I have a friend who is a Cherokee Medicine Man. His vision has been to take the most sacred part of his Native American heritage and to conduct sweat lodges for others not of his tradition, in order to share the Love he feels for the Earth and the wisdom of his culture. This is his way of growing spiritually. Each of us can also examine our own lives and see where there are opportunities to give our Love to others.

The condition of being out of balance with our own inner power and with the God-source, I have called spiritual crisis. In order to heal, we know now that we will need to rediscover who we are and to determine what we are to do with our talents. To do these things we need to find our individual visions.

True visions are mystical occurrences—markedly lucid dreams in which we see what in our ordinary lives we are too busy to see. When we have a "vision," an experience that marks our alignment with the God-force, we are nourished and more able to identify our place in the scheme of humanity's evolving.

We can call forth visions from the God-source by invoking our sincere intention to know our purposes in life. When we are ready to say to ourselves that this matter of our lives is of such importance to us that we're willing to give some of our quality time to the pursuit of greater understanding, then we will receive answers. When we try, it seems the Universe returns the gift. This universal response is perhaps what we think of as "grace." We receive insight and comfort in response to our well-directed, purposeful efforts. If we feel as if we are currently stalled in our efforts to redirect our lives, then the place to begin is at the spiritual energy level. We may not have realized it, but we are asking for a vision. This means we need to put effort at the level where answers of this sort are forthcoming: the spiritual. When we invoke the power of Love, we unknowingly invoke the spiritual dimension. This power has always been, and probably will always remain, the gateway to enlightenment.

## What Happens When We Have No Visions

When we have no visions, our bodies and the body of the planet are unsure whether we accept the present state of depression, grief, disease, and annihilation. When we have no visions, the inner energies of our bodies and emotions settle in quietly and begin to resist movement and change. This state of being isn't healthy or productive. Because we are in a time of change, the best thing we can do for ourselves is to accept that we are becoming different and that we are going to see ourselves, our bodies, our emotions, and our spirits differently. By doing so, we open ourselves to discover that the basis for all life is energy and that we are ready to explore the ways in which energy is the crucial expression of the essence we call life.

Having a vision implies being ready to do things differently. We are afraid when those who want to win our vote speak, for instance, of a future and yet themselves have no vision of humanity's place in alignment with, rather than in supremacy over, others and other forms of life. We sense intuitively that we must not trust those who tell us everything is all right and that we can continue as we have been doing, because in our hearts we are aware that the world and our lives are presently far from being in optimum balance.

We find ourselves continually put to the test to imagine our future and the qualities we will need to create this future. A woman told me recently that she doesn't dare to think beyond the immediate day. She's not sure she will have a house or a job tomorrow, that it's too fearful to think about what may come next. Can we afford *not* to think what will come next? Fear comes from having no plan, no internal story, to allow us to hope. No vision, in other words.

## Your Vision for a Future Really Counts

Every one of us is better off believing in a brighter future for ourselves and the planet. But is this belief ridiculous to even consider? If not, in what ways can life become different? No one would argue with the dismal state of the planet in which we currently find ourselves. Yet we do have choices, and we certainly have opportunities. New beginnings spring from our hearts, our hopes, and our willingness to get to work spiritually to align the future we want with the means required to bring people together to create it. All of us need to sort through our differences in search of a vision we share and are willing to make the order of the day.

Change may be slow, but it comes. We get discouraged when we think nothing is changing and the future will only be worse, but we would do well to remember that any learning curve has serious dips, times when it seems that nothing will change. When we do gradually assimilate new information, the indicators begin to rise in a positive direction. Our visions are, therefore, important to our collective future. When we share a vision of a peaceful planet in which all peoples have enough of the essentials, for instance, we are bringing the "energy," the spiritual force, of this wish ever closer to reality. The collective force of change around the world has already brought down many of the symbols of oppression that we assumed were impervious to change. Witness the removal of the Berlin wall, the dismantling of the Soviet Union as a superpower, and the breakdown of apartheid in South Africa.

Our personal visions encourage progress for humanity. And the more willing we are to work on behalf of our visions, the closer they become to reality.

## Helping Your Vision Emerge

Living a spiritual philosophy is the purpose of our lives. But we must first decide for ourselves what we can accept and what we cannot. Truth shows itself to each of us in ways that are most appropriate. So we are charged with finding and living our own truth—living Love that is the opportunity for us to grow into our greatest potential while at the same time maintaining the balance of the God-source. Certain time-honored paths lead to greater God-awareness. Several of these that I've found important and encourage you to work with are: meditation and prayer, use of spiritual language in our daily lives, ritual and ceremony to encourage direct contact with the God-source, and paying attention to the dreams, visions, insights, and teachings that come from these efforts.

When we enter into ways of celebrating our relationship with the Divine and seeking greater insight and wisdom, all the means we choose further our understanding of our own life purposes and the parts we are to play in the drama of present-day living. While much has been written about the following spiritual practices and symbologies, the perspectives

and insights offered here are steps toward these doorways to
the God-source. They deserve serious consideration.

## Meditation and Prayer

In whatever way we practice meditation, we are allowing
our active conscious awareness to probe beneath our mental
archives of experience and emotions to sense the deeper
inner peace of the Divine. When we practice meditation we
are committing to a discipline that takes time to learn and
benefit from. We are also willingly participating in a practice
that is a process, so the benefit we receive is measurable
more in months and years than in days.

The value of meditation is in its ability to help us touch
the great mystery of creation and bring that energy back
into our physical lives so that we can live more in harmony
with each other, with the living things around us, and with
the God-force. This process offers us the ultimate recharg-
ing and re-prioritizing for our lives.

Meditation requires a certain kind of relaxation. In meditation we touch the energy of the God-source that is within
us, and we give it permission to take us in search of greater
truth and Love, wherever that may lead. Allowing a spiritual
process to take control of our lives means that we need to be
willing to "lose control," and this can be fearful for many. Yet
being able to relax our rational perspective has many important benefits in allowing us to find the answers for which we
yearn. I've found that by suspending judgement as to
whether we are meditating in the right way, or are receiving
any guidance, or are gaining any benefit, we are able to relax.
No one way to meditate is right for everyone.

In meditation we search for an opening through our
cognitive thinking and reasoning processes into a perspec-

tive that shows us a different view of life and of death. We want to know what life means beyond what we can see of it ourselves. Meditation is the way to accomplish this. And it takes time and practice.

Assuming that you'll have meaningful meditations immediately will get you discouraged quickly. Consider that you are learning a new skill. After all, you didn't learn to read or to write the alphabet in a day or even a month. Be patient with yourself and with your mind, which may have trouble ceasing its chatter. Just move this mental chatter out of the way. Try to stay with attention on a single thought, phrase, or image. This keeps your spiritual energy focused on the gathering of energy and insight from the Universe rather than on your own thoughts.

Zen Buddhism speaks of the "beginner's mind." This means that as we seek intuitive understanding and direct relationship with the God-force, we should remain open and accepting rather than assuming and assertive. This injunction is similar to the requirements of Taoism, which speaks of "not-doing" in order to accomplish. Not-doing means that in order to accomplish anything in relationship to spiritual awareness we must assume an attitude of acceptance rather than active mental striving for accomplishment. Through not-doing we in fact "do."

The paths to God are found not through mental effort and struggle but through relaxing into a spiritual dimension that already surrounds us. All we need to do is let it rise around us and to accept that we are able to expand into states beyond what we now are familiar with.

Prayer is different from meditation, because during prayer we're asking for something. In prayer we're talking to God, and in meditation we're listening to God. We all need to develop a level of comfort with both these means of expressing our relationship with Divinity. Prayer alone, however, assumes that we are always in need of something that we are currently without. When we find ourselves always asking, we need to consider what we already have. Instead, consider, "What are the blessings that I'm already in possession of?"

## Using the Language of the Sacred

We are known and defined by our language and the symbols we use to communicate. As cultures we've created myths that tell of our earthly struggles to find God, to overcome disease and loss, to find joy and love, and to experience birth and death. It's comforting to realize that humanity has always asked the same questions and wanted the same cosmic reassurances.

Language is extremely important in our spiritual work because it reinforces our beliefs, validates our search, and confirms for others and ourselves the truth of our convictions. I find that as we learn about spirituality, we are often hesitant to share our insights for fear of being thought strange or intrusive. And yet when we are afraid to say what we think and to claim the truth that we are seeking to grasp, we squander the very energy we are trying to gather to us. Being afraid of what others will think of us is probably part of what got us into the physical and emotional imbalances from which we are presently trying to heal. We need to dare to be who we are and allow others the choice of accepting our positive energy. I've found that when I've assumed others will dismiss spirituality, I've been amazed to realize that what I'm saying may be exactly what they needed to hear or wanted to talk about. We people, after all, face the same questions and are in need of making similar decisions.

Our lives reflect the texture of our thoughts, and this texture in turn influences our culture's collective story. When we take our earthly journey seriously as a spiritual experience, we are more apt to enjoy our lives and feel content that we've engaged the full measure of what life has to offer us.

Using the language of the Sacred in our everyday conversation reinforces our intention to learn what life intends to teach us. We carry inside us the hopes and fears, desires and confusions, of all people, and when we are willing to wade into the ambivalences of life and the search for the Sacred, we also give others permission to grow and expand. Above all, we bring into the present time our desire, and humanity's need, to reaffirm a relationship with the God-force.

## Rituals and Ceremonies

We often feel the closest to God and the ecstasy of Divine revelation when we gather with friends and family to share the Divine through ceremony. Some examples of ceremonial characteristics we respond to are: the pomp and circumstance of a royal coronation; the incense, stained glass windows, statues, and sacred robes of a High Mass; the chanting and dancing in costume of those participating in a Native American ceremony; or the silent prayers of those gathered at a meeting of the Society of Friends (Quakers). We need ritual and ceremony in our lives.

If the truth be told, most people feel the most strongly drawn to God by the accoutrements of spirituality, those things that accompany prayer and worship. In most cultures, music is important in worship. Many people are touched, for instance, by the Hallelujah Chorus of Handel's *Messiah*. Sound and atmosphere are also important. Participants sitting in a tight circle inside an earthen hut, a sweat lodge, perform a ceremony designed to release fears through prayer, invocation, and chanting. We respond to the healing atmosphere of chants, songs, and dance performed in praise of life and the Earth.

Rituals and ceremonies are important because, even though we speak to God through our own hearts, we need others to share our experiences of revelation. So find friends who share your specific spiritual interests, and try new ways of experiencing God. The same quiet inner thought, "Let me experience what can draw me closest to a true understanding and appreciation of the God-force and keep me safe in my efforts," is all you need to keep you aligned and protected for your own greatest good.

Rituals unite our family, friends, and the entire living community through a shared desire to find harmony, peace, and loving relationships. When we participate in ceremonies and rituals that are passed down through our cultures, we wear the garments of our ancestors and re-experience their search for God. Our worship ties us to the spiritual traditions of our people and opens those time-honored pathways between heaven and Earth and the diversity of the people gathered to honor the Divine.

## Invoking the Dream State

People learn from their dreams, whether or not they are able to reconstruct them after waking up. Each night we are not just sleeping in our beds, we are being taught by the Universe. This means that we are being exposed to the ideas and spiritual truths that we can then explore in our meditations. Some dreams tell of the future, others perhaps of our past and the learning from earlier experiences. We're not limited in our dreams to any specific time or space reality. We may explore new dimensions and experience the world of spirit that, if we can remember it, might help us with our daily fears and losses. I find it helpful, before falling asleep, to put in my mind a question, need, or specific aspect of interest. Doing that enables me to travel into other realms of consciousness and seek solutions instead of spending a night tossing and turning, struggling to solve the pressing issues of daily life.

The living of a sacred reality is all around us: when we sleep, daydream, imagine, hope, pray, and meditate. It seems reasonable that the physical reality that we think is so palpable may be only a glimmer in an otherwise spiritual expression. Our visions are the bridge between the two worlds.

## The Door Is Opened

The Universe helps awaken our questions as well as our answers. In 1980 I experienced a vision that did this for me by opening a door where I was unaware that a door even existed. The Universe adds energy to our pursuit of wisdom and positive change. Once we realize that questions involving our relationships with life, with people, with the Earth, and with the God-force are all potential paths toward spiritual balance and renewed joy, then the Universe can speak with us more directly. We must take the first step before the Universe can take the second.

We've journeyed through this book together, and it seems only fitting that, as you find and share your vision with family, friends, and other spiritual seekers, I should share mine with you. Our visions are windows into ourselves at the same time they are windows into humanity's collective future. My vision is, therefore, perhaps our joint vision, because it gave me a glimpse of a possible future of humankind and spurred me to consider our choices. It was a vision of enormous hope as well as despair, with the choice resting ultimately with me and with all of us. Beyond my wildest imagination, it changed my perspective and my life irrevocably.

## The Vision that Changed My Life Forever

We tend to think we know what is true, and we tend to trust what has form. We think the familiar physical world is indestructible regardless of the words of caution now echoed by indigenous peoples, scientists, and mystics alike. I, too, felt preoccupied with the immediacy of my own needs and my family and wasn't prepared to take on a spiritual search. But the Universe isn't concerned with the limitations we've imposed on our lives. The Universe is intent upon offering us an expansive view of the truth beyond any human limitations.

My vision occurred in response to an experiment I was participating in about expanding consciousness through listening to subliminal sounds that could produce dramatic effects by balancing the left and right hemispheres of the brain. I found myself in this situation by "accident." But, of course, there are no accidents, although we may not realize that at this time.

I believe also that we are always in the places and with the people we need to be with when the next step of our spiritual journey is to unfold. And this was without a doubt my next step. I was lying down, with eyes closed, in a dark sound chamber, listening to ocean waves beneath which were subliminal sounds meant to offer the brain a chance to align its impulses synchronously. Researcher Bob Monroe, at the Monroe Institute for Applied Science in Faber, Virginia, had discovered that when yogis could hold their breath for extended periods of time, or "die" and come back, or when a person was healed by being touched by a healer, the brain impulses on both sides of the brain fired synchronously, or in exact harmony. Normally, the left and right sides of the brain fire their impulses asynchronously, or outside this harmony.[2] The subliminal sounds I was being exposed to apparently allowed for the alignment of the impulses in my own brain.

What slowly came into focus on the inner screen of my mind was a series of vivid pictures that began innocuously enough, with scenes depicting buildings in a contemporary metropolitan city—the setting could have been in New York, San Francisco, Rome, London, or Madrid. I marveled at the sleek and streamlined skyline, a tribute to humankind's technological accomplishments. Then, as if I were watching time-lapse photography, the skyline of buildings began to crumble as if dynamited from the inside. Mysteriously, helplessly, I saw the bricks and mortar of human invention and toil fell toward the ground. I watched, feeling somehow detached from the normal fear and panic that would have resulted.

The bodies, arms, and legs of people from all races slid in macabre patterns and designs across my gaze, disconnected from faces and spirits. There was no sound. I heard no scream, no cry, no plea for more time; all was silent. It was as if I stood outside the Earth, suspended like a spectator from another world, witnessing mass destruction of the familiar products of humankind's certainty.

As these images faded, a new picture began to take shape. A large and lush field of living, growing, and thriving greenness materialized in front of me. So closely were the plants growing that no soil was even visible. The ener-

gy and essence of life sprang forth as far as the human eye
could see. This plantation of interwoven foliage became a
vast and handsome carpet of life, pronouncing its presence
as if in defiance of the forces that had previously taken
away human life. In witnessing this scene, I seemed to
hover only inches above the lush expanse and yet was
aware that this proclamation of life extended beyond the
view of the human eye.

I felt this emergence of life as I had not felt the earlier
view of the loss of life. I felt at once reunited with this
scene of emerging vitality—a feeling of bursting forth from
some unseen constraints to welcome it. These living things
were my brothers and sisters, mutual journeying compan-
ions marching in row after row of joyful succession. Regret-
fully, this image, too, gradually faded.

The final aspect of this vision now emerged into my
awareness. We often speak longingly of a spiritual home, a
"place" or "space" beyond the pain, loss, and struggle of life, an
arena where all is well and where we are able to understand
and recognize our eternalness. The reality of my life, those
aspects of myself that I had identified as myself, slowly parted,
giving way to a cosmic crack between the world I knew and
that of spirit. The part of my being that could live beyond the
physical reality rose through this crack on colors of perfection.
I drifted upon a golden light out of my body, out of my life, out
of this Earth, upward, outward, or inward, to a space that was
beyond time, or maybe between times, or even between the
cycle of life and death. And I knew this was home—a new-
found dimension beyond physical life. The emotional gut-
wrenching sobs I heard my body making didn't in any way
interfere with the on-going experience as the golden glow gave
way to a vast vision of perfect clarity and pure-white calmness
extending in every direction. Like looking through the cumu-

lous clouds of all eternity, I could see forever, and it was all in place—peaceful, ordered, and beyond description.

I'm sure the experience lasted only minutes or even seconds, but the metaphor for life was clearly present, as was the metaphor for death and destruction. While I've spent years considering these images, you the reader may have your own interpretation of them. For me, this was a warning of sorts—a vision of our future and of the possibilities for our life.

I know that life is sacred, and to live with any other belief defiles life on every level. I know that physical life is only a temporary image that can vanish as quickly as it came, that a force greater than our own prevails, and that loss of life is ultimately only a circle leading back to life. Our expectation of finding a Divine home is appropriate, and our conviction that we will discover this place (or nonplace) is based on reality. Every person who has ever experienced his or her own vision in any way forever holds the certainty that there is a spiritual "home," a dimension beyond our physical reality that is eternal.

## Glimpsing Possibilities and Truth

The three parts of my vision form a circle. Who is to say which is the first and which is the last of these three parts? The fact that the aspect dealing with destruction and physical change was the first of the three sets of images seems to me to be a statement of sorts about our life on Earth and our assumptions about it. Either as an actuality or as a metaphor for change, the images of destruction certainly suggest that we are wavering on the brink of critical times. Without doubt, we are in spiritual crisis. Evolution is propelling us toward spiritual solutions that involve our willingness to accept and use Love as the energy of encouraging each person to reach his or her greatest potential.

The second aspect of the vision dealt with a carpet of vital growing life that to me suggested two important consequences of our self-indulgent culture. First, nature will ultimately survive humanity and return to a state of abundance. And second, in our arrogance we have been unwilling to accept that the relationship between nature and humanity is one unbreakable link. If in the short term we are on a path of destroying nature, in the long term we are, without doubt, destroying humanity.

Finally, the third aspect of the vision chronicled a metaphorical, or perhaps actual, but certainly inevitable, return to the realm of spirit. Not a heaven, a place of final resting, but a place of respite and of solace; perhaps a place or an inner space of spirit between lifetimes, one that allows us to reclaim a broader perspective on our physical sojourns on Earth. Until the occurrence of this vision, I never gave much thought to the question of an actual spiritual dimension of life. Like most people today, I want to believe that a spiritual "home" does exist, to trust that something does live beyond the grave. And now I am certain that it does.

The visions we are given by the Universe are a priceless gift and blessing to encourage our spiritual journey. Visions also give us the courage to speak our truth and wisdom to the community of our fellow humans in order that our shared visions can unleash energy toward a new way of living. By sharing our visions we can collectively experience the merger of all clear and decisive expressions of each person's and each culture's truth.

Sharing visions, then, is a vital part of the journey through spiritual crisis. Our march into and through the dark night of the soul is meant to break down our lives in order that we can realign them with the essential life-supporting systems of the natural world, accepting the realization of our oneness with all peoples and all living things. And finally, it is meant to show us that our shift in beliefs comes from a shift at the most basic level of beliefs—that the crack in our reality exposes us anew to the reality of the spirit and its alignment with Divinity.

My unexpected and extraordinary experience is probably an experience similar to that of many people, each slightly different but each suggesting that we walk a tightrope in life between the physical and spiritual worlds. We can have a razor's-edge experience, we can know the Sacred even though we haven't lived a monastic life, because the influence of spirit is everywhere, in everyone. The important conclusion seems to be that as we enter this apocalyptic time in our history, we are each drawn into spiritual crisis in order to metaphorically or even actually let go of physical reality as we perceive it in order to gain the realization of life as it can be on this planet and beyond. And through this experience we find, in between the worlds, the crack that leads "home."

## We Are Being Guided

We may or may not know our specific purposes or the full implication of our visions. But our visions will continue to press on our thoughts with internal questioning until we allow them to surface and guide our lives. Native peoples believed that each person was to have a vision, and that this vision guided that person in his or her Earthly endeavors. Today, we also seek to be of service to the planet and to make a meaningful contribution by our lives' effort and work.

Our visions and the fulfillment of those visions await our growth and willingness to try. We cannot determine the ways in which our visions will unfold, whether in one experience or more slowly, over an extended period of time. We can assume only that we are being guided and that our visions are awaiting us to further define themselves as we ask, question, and devote time to learning about them.

Accepting rationally that there is a Higher Power, or God, or Divine Source, and that we do fit in some way with this larger system, is very different from accepting spiritually that all life is energy and the very thoughts we put into the future create it. Knowing that our spirits are immortal is different from assuming that our culture and physical reality are. When we accept that there is more to life than we see in physical reality, and that we are to learn of these added dimensions, then the world of spiritual energy opens up before us, and we can all take serious strides toward personal and planetary healing. We are charged with aligning the energy of our thoughts with our feelings, our beliefs with our questions, and our intentions with our actions. When we are willing to consider that we are being guided toward greater understanding, then we find the blessings that our lives hold.

## Emerging from Spiritual Crisis

We are standing on an evolutionary cusp, a spur that extends into the twenty-first century, and we have enormous responsibility for more than we can ever imagine in the way of stewarding this planet and for helping each other make it better. How do we do this? Do we meditate, pray, and work on our spiritual paths? Yes, that can help! Do we protest acts of senseless destruction and violence by working to initiate actions that serve all of humanity? Absolutely! Do we direct our lives toward the living of our own highest goals? Without a doubt! Emerging from spiritual crisis, personally and planetarily, means moving beyond rationalization; we ask and expect to see life clearly. We don't want games, we want truth, and we want spiritual truth. When we hurt, we want to know why, and because we have given our lives to the living of a spiritual path, we recognize that we have a way of lessening the pain and awakening the joy.

## Creating a Healing Community

Depending upon each other is the directive for the twenty-first century. We can call on our healing coaches to help oversee our individual programs to regain energy and rebuild our bodies and emotional losses. Our healing wheels can help develop our own intimate community through which we can share and learn spiritually. And finally, the linking together of our groups, large and small, allows us to change the planet. We cannot do it alone.

Spiritual crisis is a transformative cycle tumbling us around in ways to awaken our remembered blueprint, the ways in which we are part of this planet and part of a plan for planetary transformation. This isn't so strange to consider. Spiritual crisis causes us pain, but only as we struggle to emerge as less fearful, less defensive, and less personally-needy individuals. Spiritual crisis turns us toward the light of change in ways that allow us to form alliances with those who share a vision of a healed and peaceful planet.

We are coming into a period during which many people are seeking a different way to live: a sacred path in alignment with the God-source. We are all sacred creatures of a life force we little understand. We all walk our own sacred paths—through pain and misery, loss and disease—because we are born of a spiritual energy that we want to know. We are on the Earth to experience the truth and beauty found through different ways of living, and all of this hinges on accepting a perspective based on Love.

The delineations between the layers of reality are merging. The feelings you have that spell out your own future and your own truth are but foreshadowings of the future you are creating. Just as the experimenter influences the experiment, so you influence, and are influenced by, others and by all living things. You and your spiritual energy are bonded together so that you can benefit from this extraordinary change toward a transformed planet.

## Walking the Sacred Path

Today's journey through spiritual crisis has implications that are not only personal but also communal, national, and international. Just as the personal journey through spiritual crisis is to heal our emotional losses, develop our own goodness, and initiate acts from this inner place of Love, so must nations now rise to this challenge. We can look around the planet and see the struggle for spiritual identity and awareness and the forces involved both in pushing to create a spiritual identity and in resisting these changes. Yet this global arena is the playing field on which our future success will be determined. As we near the twenty-first century, we have extremely serious inner and outer work to do as individuals in an international community.

The twenty-first century represents an evolutionary leap for humankind. The Mayan calendar ends with the year 2013, marking the beginning of a new wave of human endeavor and intention. The new century is also the awakening of the new millennium, the changeover from the astrological Piscean to the Aquarian energy. As I reflect on my own vision and the meaning it holds for today, I find that the destruction, realignment, and ascension into grace that was so vividly depicted in my vision is the model of the journey through spiritual crisis.

We can accept or reject many things about life and ourselves, but within us lies the spiritual facility for separating truth from fiction. Our inner truth is tied to a much larger and grander truth that affects every other living thing on this Earth and beyond. We are undoubtedly here in Earth-School to learn the ways that seem to break us apart and wither our bodies and feelings; yet our spirit emerges, the phoenix arising from the fire, and we go on.

We are not alone in our struggles; we are part of an infinite stream of life-energy that has come before and will long survive us. Still we will go on. Our planetary crisis is staggeringly immense, yet it can be healed. Our hearts, though broken, our lives, though left in exhaustion and pain, can be rebuilt. We are made with the capacity to love, to give Love, to share Love, to use Love, to renew Love. With Love we are capable of healing ourselves, our loved ones, and our Earth, for in accepting spiritual crisis as the challenge we also acknowledge that Love is the answer.

## NOTES

1. Meredith Lady Young, *Agartha: A Journey to the Stars* (Walpole, NH: Stillpoint Publishing, 1984).

2. Bob Monroe, Founder of the Monroe Institute of Applied Sciences, Faber, Virginia, 1980.

OTHER BOOKS & RESOURCES BY MEREDITH YOUNG-SOWERS
*Agartha: A Journey to the Stars  (Best-selling Classic)*
*Language of the Soul (A Workbook)*
*Agartha Personal Life-Balancing Program*
- *Communication*
- *Earth Connection*
- *Intuition*
- *Sexual and Emotional Balance*
- *Love*
- *Personal Power*
- *Spiritual Questing*

*Master Series Audio Tapes*
  *The Gift of Personal Power*
  *Hearing the Angelic Kingdom*
  *Soul Mates*

*Insight Series (2 audio tapes per set)*
  *I—Opportunities for Creating Dynamic Abundance*
  *II—Transcending Loneliness*
  *III—Living Your Life Purpose*

*Search for Wisdom Teaching Series (Audio Tapes)*
  *Co-Creation Course I: Applying Universal Principles for*
  *Self-Empowerment (An at-home workshop program)*

Meredith Young-Sowers's books can be purchased from your favorite bookstore or from Stillpoint Publishing. Her audio tapes, courses, and video are available only directly from Stillpoint.

*Write*:   Stillpoint Publishing
Meetinghouse Rd., P.O. Box 640
Walpole, NH    03608

*Call*:   603-756-9281
800-847-4014  (USA only)

Please address personal correspondence to Meredith Young-Sowers, c/o Stillpoint Publishing.

The Stillpoint Institute was founded on the belief that the universal insight we want and need to heal and sustain our lives and life on the planet comes from a deeper connection to the God-force and through our personal spiritual work.

Our commitment at the Institute is to create an effective network of individuals and groups of people who are seeking to use the spiritual energy of Love to heal and help themselves and others.

If you are iterested in learning more about Stillpoint Institute's outreach efforts and ways you can be part of this healing community, please write or call Stillpoint.

Stillpoint Institute for Life Healing
Meetinghouse Road,
P.O. Box 640
Walpole, NH 03608
603-756-9281